DISEASES

OF THE

HUMAN MIND

UVARA ISAAC U NELSON

First Published FEB. 2017

Copyright   Uvara Isaac U. Nelson
+2348053665634
+2347069119031

DEDICTATION

This book is dedicated to the Almighty God, the giver of wisdom, knowledge and understanding in abundance for putting this piece of work for humanity.

ACKNOWLEDGMENT

I do extend my profound gratitude to the following persons: My beloved wife Mrs. Susan Isaac U Nelson, I am proud and grateful for her great contributions toward the success of this book.

This acknowledgement will not be done without mentioning my big Daddy and the secret behind the success of this book, CSP Gbarale Dumnambara, and SP. Raymond Ogunjiofor for their fatherly advice and great contributions toward the success of this book. I also immensely thank DSP Cosmas C. Anyanwu, ASP Mary Ediete, ASP Salvation Amange.

Late father Mr. Ewa Effiong Uvara, my lovely mother Mrs. Bessi Enyi, Dr and Mrs. Bassey Benjamin Esu, Mr. and Mrs. Godwin Benjamin Esu, Apostle & Mrs. Evangelist Cleophas Ubong, Rev. Dr & (Pastor) Mrs. Emmanuel Ehwarior, Mr. Philip Ewa, Mr. Bassey Ifere, Mr. Emmanuel Nnawaku, Elder Ebere Ani. I am also indebted to every member of the Assemblies of God Church, Akwebulu Branch, Asaba, Delta State of Nigeria for their prayers and general supports. God bless you all.

PREFACE

This book focuses on root causes and effects of negative emotional feelings such as anger, fear, aggression, anxiety, doubt, pride, hatred and many others and how they affect our psychological, physiological and spiritual growth and development. Many people think they are healthy but are victims of psychological disorders and spiritual deformity of phobia, anger, the lack for forgiveness, doubt. These conditions herein referred to as "Diseases of the Human Mind" are more toxic than the physical ailments.

This book however, is dedicated to proffer solution to these negative emotional feelings that affect us, our relationship with God as well as our fellow human beings. It also contains practicable approaches that include prevention and solution, moment of introspection (sober reflection), and ways to strengthening our relationship with God and humanity.

The focus is to structure our minds and mindset for self evaluation, connecting with cosmic nature, self control, developing a positive healthy lifestyle of extraordinary and divine dynamism and empowerment.

CONTENTS

1. Page Title
2. Dedication/Acknowledgment
3. Preface
4. Contents

CHAPTER 1:   INTRODUCTION

CHAPTER 2:   THE HUMAN MIND

CHAPTER 3:   ANXIETY

CHAPTER 4:   FEAR

CHAPTER 5:   DOUBT

CHAPTER 6:   ANGER

CHAPTER 7:   ENVY/JEALOUSY

CHAPTER 8:   UNFORGIVENESS

CHAPTER 9:   PRIDE

CHAPTER 10:   HEALING THE MIND

CHAPTER   11:   MOMENT   OF   SOBER
                    REFLECTION

CHAPTER 1
INTRODUCTION

The human mind is the originality of man, If you want to manipulate him, hold on to his mind. If you want him to talk more, just hold on to his mind and stir it to the point that he will start talking.

Man's interpretation of God's mind through His word has resulted to the injury of his fellow man. This has resulted in many people withdrawing from God, others doubting God's authority, mercy, grace and ability. Man's relationship with God is something that has remained a point of concern in the mind of many. One thing to note is, man is a finite being while God is an infinite being. Man is not an independent product of existence; he is a dependable being. He needs the presence of God to gain true joy, happiness and lasting peace. Until this is realized, the gap between him and his creator will continue to erode. His continue learning and discovery will only bring him confusion, languish in pains, regrets, confusion and frustration of the mind. Like I earlier said, every individual needs to realize that he is a creation- a product of God's idea, wisdom, and handwork and come to term that there is a creator (God) who owns everything about him. His **spiritual and physical growth and success** therefore, depends largely on the extents of his relationship with his creator.

This relation is established in a place called the **mind**; you can call it the heart of man. Andrew M. Coleman (2003) described it as the "***soul***". The Greek word called it "***Psyche***". It is the foundation or the only avenue where you can see God. Matthew 5:8 says blessed are the **pure in heart**: for they shall see God. It can also be described as the ***battle ground of man's life***. Inside this place called mind, is a place that cannot be directly measured or access but by some observable characteristics of our emotional reactions.

One thing that has remains unnoticed in the House of God is the expression of the emotional feelings. A whole lot of people go to church with spiritual and psychological burdens in their minds. It is unfortunate to say that many still go home with those burdens right inside their minds unsolved. Even in the face of powerful messages been preached, they still remain the same or even worst. The secret of this problem lies within our minds. Since we cannot observe directly or measure the contents of the human mind, we can measure them through the expression of our emotional feelings such as fear, anger, excitement, aggressiveness, bodily reaction, joy, happiness, sadness and many more. These characteristics are the elements that portray our behaviors. Show me a healthy man, I will show you a man who is happy within his mind. On the other hand, show me a sick man and I will show you a man with his mind riddled with fear, anxiety, anger, frustration, confusion, hatred, lack of forgiveness, bitterness and internal pains.

These expressions enable us to communicate our feelings to other people and also regulate how other people respond to us, (Izard-1989, 1991). The similarity of facial expression across culture exemplifies the communication function of emotions. Our emotions reflect the same way we feel. Our emotions are non observable behavior which can be measured by the way we feel and are usually accompanied by physiological reaction, (J.G Carlson and Hatfield, 1992). For instance, when you see a man who is sad, you will notice his facial expression, bodily reaction and even his speeches. Similarly, one who is happy of course will be easier to tell. Example of emotional feelings includes joy, sadness, happiness, anger, fear, transfer aggression, anxiety, doubt, pride, love, hatred and many others.

Another basic fact about these negative emotional feelings which I termed here as: **diseases of the mind,** is that they have the power to suppress the individual emotionality to such an extent that he no longer gets control of his original state of mind. In fact, they are the center focus of this book. Further to say that, it takes a very few seconds to activate them but it take a very long time to restore the mind (soul) after the body become tensed when these diseases are triggered. This is also applicable to the extent of damages they could cause to our bodies. In my own observation and conclusion, the spiritual damages or harm caused by these diseases are far more fatal and destructive than the physical assessment. Proverbs 14:13 made it clear; "A sound mind is the life of the flesh." This indicates that the flesh or body is solely dependent on the mind.

If I may ask, is there any fact saying that anger, pride, fear, doubt, murmuring, pride, hatred, jealousy/envy promote or enhance our relationship with God and man? Charles Darwin once argued that all people express certain basic feeling in the same way without knowing a person language- The Expression of the Emotion in Man and Animal (1872).

THE CONCEPT OF THE MIND

The human mind is a cognitive faculty that enables consciousness, perception, judgment, and memory. The human mind is such an intellectual concept and a complex one indeed. Sigmund Freud and William James during the 21st century developed various approach to the understanding of the human mind. This concept is understood in many cultures and religions. Many writers believe that love, hatred, fear, anxiety, anger etc. are subjective; other theorists argued that these emotional concepts cannot be separated from the mind.

The human mind is also formed from series of learning processes. Overtime, this accumulated experiences form a belief that is enshrined in his mind. This learning concept determines the structure of the mind. According to John Locke, **the human mind is empty at birth**. It is during the process of growth; that we skill, knowledge, understanding, evil and good and many other things. The human mind is like a city, the buildings and structure in it are determined by the owner of the city. Likewise, your mind, you determine its structure and functionality by what you acquire. The type of community setting determines the type of people within its environment. The type of persons we have in our community is determined by our mindsets. This also affects the psycho-social behavior of the individual. If an individual finds himself in a locality where the resources are limited, such an individual's mind will become narrow and limited to the tools required for the journey of life. You acquire those tools that help shape as well as the functionality of your mind by developing a positive self concept, self esteem, effective and efficient learning processes, and association with different type of personalities.

The human mind is the originality of the man. It is the life of the individual. If you take it away from him, he is dead. This is what determines his personality (the sum total of the psychological, physical and spiritual description of his real self). This personality structure is formed and guided by principles, what to do, what not to do, the good and the bad that define who he is. That is where you hear people describing him as good or bad person. This concept in summarily is described as the "mindset".

What you acquire becomes part of you; I mean your personality (spiritual and physical). If you acquire what is good, then your mind will radiates positivity, but if you acquire evil, your mind becomes evil. This is where we talk about faith and mindset. Faith is the substance of things hoped for, the evidence of things not seen (Hebrew 11:1).

Faith is the belief of the unseen with a high expectation. **Faith can also be described as a principle of the mind** that enables the individual keep to what he believes in. Faith is not of the body. It connects you to the cosmic nature. Faith also helps you connect to the unseen future and what is contained in it. Without faith the future is meaningless and nonexistence. We have never seen the future but faith transport us to the future. One thing you must understand is that between you and the future is a dark path. It takes men of vision and faith to see through this dark path in other to excel through. When the Psalmist understood it, he said Yea, **though I walk through the valley of the shadow of death** (the dark path to success), I will fear no evil: for thou art with me; thy rod and thy staff they comfort me. The Psalmist was connecting faith with the content of his mind (fear). In other word, if I want to truly walk through the valley of the shallow of death, I need two things- "**faith**-connecting God" and "**my mind**- believing myself). God has prepared ...... anointed my head. This is the expression of faith in action. **Faith therefore helps you hold tight to what your mind perceived**. When faith grows to its full height it become faithfulness, or put it the fullness of faith. If in your mind, there are elements of trust that there is a living God, then your mind will grasp this belief never to let it go. This is what we called **Faith**. Faith therefore, becomes that substance that helps you as a person to focus your vision on what you believe and never let it go. Faith empowers your mind to walk through the dark path of life. You cannot be vision focus with a well developed mindset of faith and remain where you are even years after. Faith repositions you. Faith serves as a transitional force. Your faith in God is what determines your position in God. Your faith in God will not give any chance to the devil to take control of your mind. Faith enshrined in the mind helps you get focus and determination. This is where 20 Acts:19 advised us saying **"Serving the LORD with all humility of mind, and with many tears, and temptations, which befell me by the lying in wait of the Jews."**

We can never mention the human mind without mentioning the mindset. Your mindset is the composition and structure of your mind. It is the sum total of your self-concept, learning outcome, thinking patterns, actions, ideologies and perception which are both physical and spiritual. Your mindset is the total magnum opus of your mind. Your mindset is what determines your belief system, your personality and behavioral patterns. Your mindset also influences your level of faith. Your mindset is also determined by the level of your faith. These two variables are inseparable. You cannot take faith from your mindset. A weaker mindset influences a weaker faith. A well formidable mindset influences a substantial faith. A God-designed faith also determines a potentials mindset.

It is also significant to note that a man may have a thousand enemies but the worst enemy here is always the disintegration of his mind. This is because when an external factor attacks you, you can still stand and have sense of unity within you (mind and body). But when you are at conflict with your mindset, your personality (body and mind) becomes disorganized, disunited, and separated from his creator (God). You become disoriented and psychologically jumbled. At this point, you immediately begin to lack focus and concentration, confusion and pessimism begin to occupy his mind. Most people begin to transfer the contents of their mind (frustration, confusion, anger, sadness, gloomy etc) to other people. This is what psychologists called defense mechanism- a negative means to discharge negativity and/or protecting the self. The Psalmist says "many are the afflictions of the righteous: but the LORD delivered him out of them all." Others discharge their anger/frustration on food, drinks, sex, sleep, reading, wives, friends, relatives, watching movies and/or animal. In most cases, you hear people telling you "I just need some time"; "please I do not need any disturbances." Loneliness sometimes becomes their comfort.

In worst, scenario most people develop to chronic depression, suicidal thoughts and suicide becomes the end result. It is not the physical war but the war of the mind riddled with anger, confusion, jealously, fear, doubt, disgust, anxiety and many others. That is the reason a boss comes to the office sadden, angered, depressed, frustrated and set his office on fire. A man wakes up depressed and confused, and then gets angry with every person in the house. He gets to the church and come out the same and/or even worst.

This is where Paul in Roman 7:23 described the human mind as a battle ground "**But I see another law in my members, warring against the law of my mind, and bringing me into captivity to the law of sin which is in my members.**" Martin Luther King, speech, Aug. 16, 1967 had this to say "As long as **the mind is enslaved**, the body can never be free. Psychological freedom, a firm sense of self-esteem, is the most powerful weapon against the long night of physical slavery". The battle of the mind is the greatest battle of all time. This is because his **mind is the master power that moulds, makes, or even destroys him**.

QUOTES FROM HEROES

The mind grows by what it feeds on. **JOSIAH GILBERT HOLLAND**, Lessons in Life.

The mind commands the body and immediately it obeys. The mind orders itself, and meets resistance. **BRIAN HERBERT & KEVIN J. ANDERSON**, The Butlerian Jihad.

CHAPTER 2
THE HUMAN MIND

If you want to manipulate a man hold on to his mind. If you want him to talk more just hold on to his mind and stir it to the point that he will start talking

The Webster's Dictionary defines the human mind as the element in an individual that feels, perceived, think, wills and especially reason.

The human mind has the following key characteristics:

> The Human mind is cosmic. It is the central point or element in man that has celestial nature and which enable him communicate with the unseen nature.

- The human mind is the seat of ideation, memory, visions, critical thoughts, insight and visualization.
- The human mind is also the central point which enables him transcends into the world beyond. This is enhanced through effective and consistent prayers and meditation.
- The human mind is dynamic and progressive. Romans 12:2, "…. but be ye **transformed** by the **renewing of your mind**, that ye may prove what is that good, and acceptable, and perfect, will of God". Ephesians 4:23, said "…. **be renewed** in the spirit of your mind".

THE TWO NATURE OF THE HUMAN MIND

The Positive or the Spirit Man: The positive man is characterized by a mindset that promotes healthy life style of the individual and the society. The positive mind sees life as a gift and seeks the good and progress of the society. This positive mindset bears fruits which include joy, love, peace, longsuffering, gentleness, goodness, faith, meekness, temperance. The spirit man is always in the spirit and operates in a positive attributes. It is well organized, dynamic, well thought-out and always guarded against selfishness, competitiveness and self-centeredness, pride, vain glory, provoking and envying one another. He is guided by Philippians 4:8- meditate and set your mind therein.

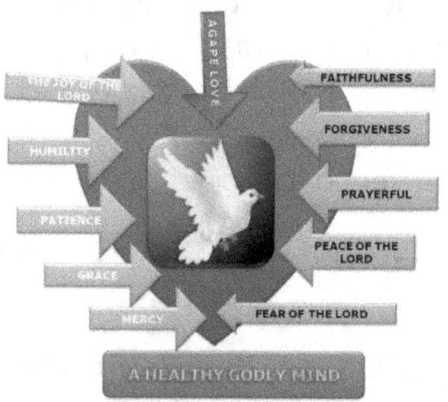

The Negative or the Fleshy Man: The negative or fleshy man operates in the flesh. He is characterized by selfishness, egoism, worldly desire of materialism, I-want-all syndrome and avariciousness which include

Adultery, fornication, uncleanness, lasciviousness, Idolatry, witchcraft, hatred, variance, emulations, wrath, strife, seditions, heresies, Envying, murders, drunkenness, drugs addicts, homosexuality, medium practice, reveling, and such like. The fleshy man is self-principle oriented. It has nothing good for others rather it is designed to take from others.

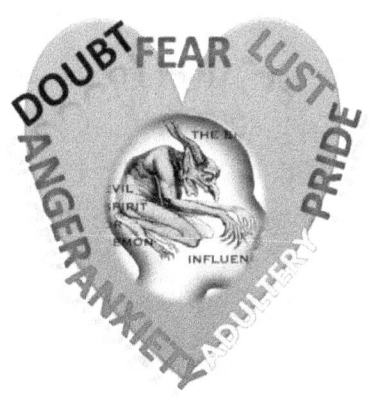

These two natures of the human mind are what determine your mindset. They are the foundations of your mindset. Your mind is the foundation upon which your personality is structured. They guard you to make decisions, take actions and chose between what is right or wrong. Mindset therefore is defined as a complex mental state involving beliefs, feeling, values, judgments, morality, opinions, thoughts, principles and positions to act in a certain ways.

Mindset can also be seen as the totality of what the mind perceived, grasp and become part of the mind. In a fixed mindset, people believe their basic qualities, like their intelligence or talent, are simply fixed traits. Most people have their mindset structured from Biblical point of view. Others have their mindset structure from what happened to them. To some, it is structure base on mental perception of life or circumstances of life.

Another aspect of the human mind is the mind at conflict. This stage is characterized by disintegration of the mind following indecision, lack of concentration of the self and internal conflict of judgment. There is a struggle of evil and good with the individual. People characterized with this problem do not go to war. Two things will likely happen; it is either they die half way or they help kill their partners or leader. These types of people easily betray their leaders in tough time.

THE MIND AND THE BODY

Aristotle believed the mind and the body are one and same *(monism).* Plato believed the mind is located within the body but are different from each other *(Body-Mind Dualism)*. Hippocrates also believed or considered the location of the mind to be within the body- (ca. 428-348 BC.) In Rene Descartes' opinion, the human mind and its power are supreme: *Cognito ergo sum* (Latin word for "I think therefore I exist". According to him, the mind influences the body.

The Bible rightly put it, **as a man think** that is who he is. This implies that the outcome of your thought and ideation determines the course of your actions. That is why **if you want to manipulate a man hold on to his mind. If you want him to talk more**

just hold on to his mind and stir it to the point that he will start talking. If you want him to see God, begin to fill his mind with the word and reposition his mind to a frequency where he will begin to see and understand that God is talking. **If you want to reposition a man's behavior, first reposition his mind.** Whatever you want him to do, start from his mind. The devil understands this secret, so he has nothing to do with your body. He is concern with your mind. Though, he uses things of the flesh to gain access to your mind. That is why your mind is the center focus for the devil. The devil manipulated Eve's mind by just placing the idea of the forbidden fruit in her mind. He did not force her. It was just a suggestion presented to her. Eve's mind captures it and did the rest. Our minds are like a fertile ground. It never rejects any seed of thought at first instance, except you quickly understand the nature and purpose of that seed in your mind.

That is the reason the Bible speaks so much about the human mind. Jesus made mention of the human mind much more than the body. In Luke 10:16-17, after he cast out demon from a dumb person, the Pharisees and Sadducees decided to tempt him in their mind. Jesus quickly understood the content of the mind. The Bible said, he (Jesus) knowing their thoughts (content of the mind) *power of thoughts and ideation*. Your mind is the production center for ideas and thoughts irrespective of your conscious effort. Eighty percent of your ideas and thoughts are involuntary whether you are asleep or not. These thoughts are unconsciously generated from within our mind. We grab and make use of very few ones while others vanish without any human effort.

Jesus Christ during his earthly ministry was so particular about the human mind much more than their actions because He understood the power house of man than man himself. See Mark 2:6-8. The Bible will always describe Jesus' respond as **"knowing their thoughts" (The Good News Bible), New King James Version** put it this way,

"Jesus Perceived". It is pertinent to note that wrong decisions damage your mind faster and easier but right decisions may be hard to come by but keeps you formidable and alive. **Your mind is the candle of the LORD**, searching all the inward parts of the belly- Proverbs 22:27. In Proverbs 21:1, "The Lord controls the **MIND** of a King as easily as he directs the course of a stream. Do you know that your "**mind is the temple of God within you which you have from God, you are not your own**- I Cor. 6:19". God's temple must be Holy. For the human mind to be the dwelling place or God's temple, then the human mind must be holy. For the human mind to be holy, it must be guarded to accommodate the spirit of God. For the human mind to be God's dwelling place, first **you must allow** him to take possession. You must sanctify it to accommodate the Holy Spirit. That is the reason Christ once said, I stand at the door and knock, those who recognize him, allow Him to come in. The truth of the matter is that your mind determines who you are, what you do, and how you do it. You have to bear in mind that **one iota of a successful thought can make you a winner**. On the other hand, **one atom of any wrong thought can paves way to failure in life**. These thoughts are originated within your mind.

Like I earlier said, you must note that the mind is the center for thought. This thought could be **good** or **evil** depending on **who possesses that mind**. When Paul was talking about the mind in Philippians 2:5, "he said having this mind (**the mind of God**) among yourselves which is in Christ Jesus". Paul was advising the Philippians' Christian brothers to be of **one mind (a unified state of mind).** He emphasized strongly on virtues that will admonish and renew their minds, "if there be anything ……. put your mind on those things (feed your mind with those things) –

Philippians 4:8 says "Finally, brethren, whatsoever things are true, whatsoever things are honest, whatsoever things are just, whatsoever things are pure, whatsoever things are lovely, whatsoever things are of good report; if there be any virtue, and if there be any praise, **think on these things**

(Feed your mind on those things)".

It is also very important to note that when you become a new man, it is not the body that becomes transformed; it is the human mind (***psyche***) which is the core and power house that gets transformed. You become a new man because your mind is liberated from the bondage of limitation and regains its original creation. You become new because the devil leaves your mind, and give way to the Holy Spirit. At this point, your ideation, thought, perception, mentality takes a new turn. The way you perceive things takes a new dimension. Your perception takes a new dimension. You begin to see the universe from a new dimension of beauty and positivity. This is because you are now in line with the reality of life unlike those living in the shadow of others. Your mind will begin to identify and reject evil because it realizes that evil is toxic. In the next chapter we are going to examine some of the diseases and how they affect us spiritually, physically and psychologically.

DISEASES OF THE MIND

Disease according to Longman Dictionary of Contemporary English (The Living Dictionary) is defines as something that is seriously wrong with someone's mind, behavior etc. Diseases of the human mind in this contexts is defines as any emotional or psychological and spiritual ailment or disorder that disrupt the functionality of the individual's spiritual and psychological development and growth.

These diseases include those that affect not only the individual as a person but the community as a whole. This includes anxiety, fear, anger, envy, doubt, Adultery, fornication, uncleanness, lasciviousness, Idolatry, witchcraft, hatred, variance, emulations, wrath, strife, seditions, heresies, envying, murders, drunkenness, drugs addicts, homosexuality, medium practice, reveling etc. in this context however, we are going to discuss some which are predominant and are seen as basic to the survival of an average individual.

These diseases are far from what you think. If there is any deadly disease you can ever think of, then think of anxiety, fear, doubt, envy/jealousy, pride and the lack of forgiveness ... Then you will understand better. These diseases are contagious and communicable. We hardly noticed how people with fear disorder affect our lives. This is applicable to those with anxiety, anger, pride, hatred and the spirit of unforgiveness.

There never can be a man so lost as one who is lost in the vast and intricate corridors of his own lonely mind, where none may reach and none may save- **ISAAC ASIMOV, Pebble in the Sky.** There is nothing mind can do that cannot be better done in the mind's immobility and thought-free stillness- **SRI AUROBINDO, Essays Divine and Human**

CHAPTER 3
ANXIETY

Each day has its task. It takes special people and men of courageous mind like you to scale through the roughness of life. Life is a battle ground; nothing good comes easy in life. You must fight for it.

A typical human being faces the battles of sorrow, misery and worry on a daily basis. Many others are confronted with the challenges of tackling fear, stress, and anxiety. With the world running on the fast lane of materialism and hunger for achievement, yet many are consistently crashing on daily basis. Others are afraid to crash on the same path of life. So they are all doing all they can to avoid running on that rock of life. Anxiety has not only remained an individual problem but the community, organization, the government and a global disorder. Despite all these anxieties, we have succeeded in achieving nothing except filling our cupboard with drugs to combat anxiety. The modern man only discovered that he unknowingly created anxiety for himself after ignoring or trying to modify nature to fit his demands or needs. He invented so much to comfort himself and did so little to manage the after effect of his discoveries. So he became afraid of what he invented for himself. He also misunderstood and misapplied what Genesis 1:28 said "... be fruitful, and multiply, and replenish the earth, and subdue it: and **have dominion** over the fish of the sea, and over the fowl of the air, and over every living thing that moves upon the earth. He discovered so much, he invented so much, he traded so much, enriched himself with so much but had very little control of all these achievement which are now his source of anxiety. He hardly sleeps comfortably due to tomorrow's worries of the unknown.

Corrie ten Boom once said "Worrying is carrying tomorrow's load with today's strength- carrying two days at once. It is moving into tomorrow ahead of time. Worrying does not empty tomorrow of its sorrow, it empties today of its strength. I have always noticed that people with anxiety disorder seem to focus much on the future with so much little concentration on the present. That is why their foundation for tomorrow which starts today is always shallow and baseless.

One may asked is it wrong to worry about the future or something that may bother the mind. The answer is simply no. Except when you allow abnormal anxiety without a purpose take over your mind. The reality of life is not the challenges you face but how your mind respond to these challenges. If you allow anxiety fill your mind, the only thing you will see is persistent darkness of the future. I think Augustine of Hippo was right when he said "The punishment of every disordered mind is its own disorder." We often time help our mind to develop this disorder.

THEN WHAT IS ANXIETY IN THIS CONTEXT

Anxiety is defined by Psychologists as nervous feeling caused by fear that something is about to happen or put it an **excessive state of tense,** worried, scare and anxious feeling arises from no meaningful events (Andrew Coleman 2003). Robert Sternberg (2001) defines anxiety as a **generalized feeling of dread** or **apprehension** that is not focused on or directed toward any particular object or event. Anxiety as most Bible called it **"Heaviness in the heart"** is not only a psychological disorder but a spiritual condition, which is why the Bible seriously warns against it. Matthew 6:25 put it this way; "Therefore, I tell you, do not be **anxious** about your life of what to eat, drink, wear ………". Anxiety in a man's heart is a burden but a good word gladdens him- (Proverb 12:25). The Bible advises us to be bold like a lion and stable like a mountain.

The book of Proverbs 12:25, states; Anxiety in a man's heart weight him down causing **spiritual imbalance and confusion. You cannot be bold and stable if you are riddle with anxiety**. The only thing you can accept is the disintegration and confusion of the mind followed by excessive nervousness and lack of concentration. The simple truth is this; nothing kills a man faster than a state of mind riddle with anxiety and self disturbances. Though in most cases, we feel nervous and a little bit worried. In this case however, it is normal to act that way but when we allow situations get control of our entire system (spiritual and psychosocial development) then it becomes abnormal.

Anxiety arises because we interpret a stimulus as threatening - the interpretation is more important than the actual stimulus. There are many theories that are variations and elaborations on this theme (eg: Beck & Emery, 1985; Ellis & Harper, 1976).

SYMPTOMS OF ANXIETY

- Tension
- Nervousness
- Uncomfortable arousal
- Distress
- Lack of concentration
- Excessive worry
- Sudden panic
- Sleep disorder
- Sudden anger
- Displacement of frustration
- Depression
- Confusion
- Sudden stress etc.

ANXIETY CAUSES THE FOLLOWING PROBLEMS:

Anxiety is a potential force that conditions us to doubt ourselves and our abilities. It causes us to **doubt** supernatural power and authority. No wonder many Christians and great men are running from pillar to posts seeking miracles and financial explosion yet nothing happen. Anxiety is also a potential source of spiritual malady such a prayerlessness, tempered faith, deteriorated spiritual life. Each time you feel anxious, there are tendencies that your body temperature will change. This consistent body temperature could triggers unwarranted stimulus resulting to other forms of disorders such as digestive disorder, increase in blood pressure, impaired vision, psychological stress and fatigue.

Anxiety if not properly controlled can have a serious negative effect on our mental functioning. If anxiety can cause such an enormous threat to our physical lives what about the spiritual aspect? Jesus Christ understood it and advised us not to worry for nothing. God knows what is expected of us, He knows our need and he will supply our needs according to His riches in glory. The secret is, be focused and believed him, his word and who he is. Romans 13:5 say, **"Wherefore ye must needs be subject, not only for anxiety/wrath, but also for conscience sake.** The problem of anxiety comes when we detached ourselves from our creator. In most cases, we tend to operate on our own. God said call upon me in times of trouble and I will deliver you out. One reason we suffer anxiety is disobedient to God's instruction. We become vulnerable when we neglect or reject God's instruction.

SPIRITUAL DANGERS ASSOCIATED WITH EXCESSIVE ANXIETY

1. Anxiety kills our prayer and spiritual life by injecting disbelief and doubt in us. Anxiety serves as a neutralizer of God's word and his promises to us. Depressed people always complain against God. Whosoever complaint against God or the potential power of the Holy Spirit stands the chance of barring himself from the presence of God. A disintegrated mind cannot receive blessings from God.

2. Anxiety can lead to **depression**. We become more exposed to suicidal thoughts and conclude that life has nothing good for us. Psalm 42:11 has this to say "Why art thou **cast down** (**depression**), O my soul? and why art thou disquieted within me? hope thou in God: for I shall yet praise him, who is the **health** of my countenance, and my God".

3. With depression we become more pessimistic and less optimistic. We become vulnerable to temptations of life. We tend to see a blur vision about the future and God's promises. See John 14:11-12, "**Believest thou not** that I am in the Father, and the Father in me? The words that I speak unto you I speak not of myself: but the Father that dwelleth in me, he doeth the works... Verily, verily, I say unto you, He that **believeth on me**, the works that I do shall he do also; and greater works than these shall he do; because I go unto my Father".

4. It depersonalizes our sense and makes us feel that God is not real. I earlier said that one of the characteristics of the human mind is to transcend into the cosmic. This cosmic nature is to connect with our creator. Our minds play a vital role in connecting with the Holy Spirit of God. Our inability to transcend to this cosmic nature is barred by abnormal and persistent state of anxiety.

5. Anxiety kills our physical and spiritual potentials. It makes us feel worthless,

vulnerable and more distrustful. When we become anxious for nothing, it blinds us spiritually; we hardly recognize our spiritual gifts and potentials.

6. It makes God non existence; all his promises for us become a mirage and the Bible become a mere writings or literature.

7. Anxiety can trigger other health related ailment such as headache, increase blood sugar, visual impairment etc. most of us do interpreted III John 1:2 " I wish above all things that you may **be in good health**, just as your soul prosper". If I may ask, is your psychological and physical state of health not an integral part of your spiritual health? God is concerned about your body and soul, your physical and spiritual health. Do not let anxiety mar it for you. When John the Beloved discovered this secret, he said "**I wish above all things** that thou mayest prosper and be in health, even as **thy soul prospereth**". (III John 1:2).

8. The irony of it all is that each time you worry, it does nothing good to you, and **it**

does not add any cubit to your status rather it reduces and even **destroy your brain and body cells** - Matthew 6:27. The only thing excessive anxiety can help do is to bring your untimely death faster than expected. **Charles Haddon Spurgeon** once said "Our anxiety does not empty tomorrow of its sorrows, but only empties today of its strengths." Anxiety can also help you ignore today's benefits and focus on tomorrow's problems.

9. During anxiety, we show evidence of some level of spiritual discomfort such as uncertainty, worry and even fear of nothing.

10. Anxiety can also help create some delusion fantasies against friends, and relatives. In most cases, we tend to become more apprehensive of people around us without a cause.

OTHER NEGATIVE EFFECTS OF ABNORMAL ANXIETY INCLUDE:

1. Excessive anxiety could cause brain disease or condition such as amnesia- A brain condition characterized by loss of explicit memory.
2. Anxiety could also lead to hypertension. This is because each time you are worried, your blood pressure rises. The rise of blood in the body put pressure on the heart.
3. Visual impairment and redness of the eyes are another side effect of excessive anxiety.
4. Anxiety is such a dangerous disease that can even abort pregnancy. This is because anxiety follows consistence state of psychological disturbances. This psychological disturbance can leads to physiological imbalance leading to sleep disturbance, abnormal hormonal secretion and redness of the eyes.
5. Many individuals have failed in various job interviews simply because they were anxious and disturb over nothingness.
6. Anxiety helps you trigger others negative emotional reactions such as doubt, anger,

fear. It exposes you to vulnerability. You become less protective and unsecure.

SECRET TO CONQUER ANXIETY

Rick Warren once advised that "The more you pray, the less you will panic. The more you worship, the less you worry. You will feel more patient and less pressured." The more you pray, the bolder you become. Prayer is not only a communication medium between you and God but a source of inner strength and courage. Prayer reinforces you for the battle and challenges of life. Prayer therefore remains the number therapy over anxiety. See I Thessalonians 5:7, "Pray without ceasing", James 5:15 says "And the prayer of faith shall **save the sick**, and the Lord shall raise him up; and if he have committed sins, they shall be forgiven him".

According to Hazrat Ali Ibn Abu-Talib A.S "Do not let your difficulties fill you with anxiety; after all it is only in the darkest nights that stars shine more brightly." You must learn the act of letting it go no matter how difficult it is. Each time you let it go, you off load your mind with difficulties. Instead of looking at life, look unto God through Jesus Christ the author and finisher of your faith: who for the joy that was set before him endured the cross, despising the shame, and is set down at the right hand of the throne of God." Hebrew 12:2.

You must learn how to work with your mind not your body. This is your ability to blend faith and productive and effective work. There are two set of human beings I know (a) Those who taste the fantasy of success through dreams. They are living in their dreams but never committed to productive work. These set of people are afraid to step out of faith. Most importantly, they do not commit their ways to connect with God. So they work with all their might. Proverbs 16:3 says "Commit thy works unto the LORD, and thy thoughts shall be established." (b) Those that will rather taste the reality of failure than sitting in the dark and taste the fantasy of success that will never. This people are not only riddled with fear of stepping out in faith but worried about the outcome of the unknown. This is what they say; I am worried what will happen if it does not come the way I expect.

In Psalm 139, the Psalmist understood this secret and prayed saying "search me, O God, and know my heart: try me, and know my thoughts(the contents of his mind): Thou knowest my down-sitting (weaknesses) and mine uprising (strength), thou understand my thought afar off. You must learn to connect to God's clinic on daily basis so His Holy Spirit will run some spiritual health check on your mind. You may be physically healthy but spiritual lacking. The two clinics you need to visit are God's clinic and man-made clinic. My substance was not hid from thee, when I was made in secret, and curiously wrought in the lowest parts of the earth. He knows everything about you.

Life is one step at a time. There may be thousands of problems on the ground but you will require removing one problem at a time. While you are solving each problem at a time, you must also acknowledge God with thanksgiving. Do not be anxious about the enormous problems of life, but in each step, by prayer, and petition, focus with thanksgiving, present your requests to God and He will grant you the wisdom and strength to move ahead. Each day has its task. It takes special people and men of courageous mind like you to scale through the roughness of life. Life is a battle ground; nothing good comes easy in life. You must fight for it. When you become anxious of the next task without solving the current task, you will only complicate them. When somebody tells you that life is a battle ground, it psychologically and spiritually programs you to be competitive, prayerfully aggressive, focused, courageous and optimistic. Life must not be seen from a do or die perceptive but a gift. Life is beautiful and must be enjoy to the fullest. You only need to discover the secrets of life's mysteries of connections.

Do not let your hearts be troubled and do not be afraid of the things of the world. Riches and wealth is not bad. They become evil with the absence of God when materials things occupy the mind. Life can be relatively smooth and peaceful when you cast all your anxiety on him because he cares for you.

Develop the mindset of faith and faithfulness in God. Until you dedicate your entire mindset on the things of God and stay focus on him, life itself will be miserable. You must realize that the greatest therapy for anxiety is a mindset built on God's faith. You can develop this type of faith by constantly going to places of worship and have a better and a stronger personality with God, Jesus Christ and the Holy Spirit. Feeding on the word of God is the basis for understanding and remaining focus in his presence. This book of the law shall not depart out of thy mouth; but thou shalt **meditate therein (Mind at work)** day and night, that thou mayest observe to do according to all that is written therein: for then thou shalt make thy **way prosperous**, and then thou shalt have **good success**. Joshua 1:8.

CHAPTER 4
FEAR

Fear is a mind-destroyer. Faith is a mind-builder, while fear sees the past; faith sees a bright and a successful future.

This chapter look at the various angles of fear, what causes fear, what actually are the dangers associated with fear; maybe we can check if fear is necessary at all.

If there is one dangerous barrier that can make a dream impracticable to accomplish, then think of excessive fear. When we are afraid of life, we pull back, but when we are courageous about life we push forward. A man with fear disorder is a candidate of failure but a man full of faith is a candidate of success. While fear sees the past, faith sees a successful future. People with fear look backward. Those with faith look forward. When we develop a courageous mind, we are open to every gift and beauty life has to offer us such as enthusiasm, optimism, excitement, and hope. Fear is a mind-destroyer. Faith is a mind-builder. Fear and faith are two opponents of the mind of any individual. They are at each other's neck. The absence of faith brings fear and vice versa. When we fear, we become scare but when we show faith, we attack rather than retreat. It is what you do that determine who occupies and direct the course of your mind. Your opponent can only defeat you when you show him that you are ruled by fear. In most cases the things we fear in life need only to be understood, and approach with God's kind of knowledge. The irony of it all according to **Paulo Coelho, The Alchemist** states that our deepest fear is that we are powerful beyond measure. It is our light, not our darkness that most frightens us. We are afraid that success may not get to us, so we become frightened on the ground we might fail in the end.

Fear is rooted back to the Greek word "*phobos*" meaning fear- Andrew Coleman (2003). Psychologists define fear as excessive and irrational feeling of an object, image, situation, condition of thing not seen. Many people may not understand the true meaning of fear because to them, it is just part of everyday life, not to mention it effect (psychological, psychological, and spiritual). The truth is that fear is very inimical to the developmental growth of any individual. When fear become excessive that it cannot be easily controlled or managed, it results to a condition called Phobia- from the same Greek word "***phobos***" meaning fear and "***ia***" indicating a condition. Phobia (excessive fear) is a persistent, excessive and irrational feeling that disrupt normal life situation. It could require spiritual, chemotherapeutic or psychological attention. It is very unfortunate to note that fear at its extreme level may not have accurate medical diagnosis, so guide against it.

Robert Sternberg (2001) believes people are overly sensitive to other people's judgment or when they are unable to accept their own nature. We seem to blame others for our actions. We are sometimes afraid to accept our own indecisions, omission and ignorant because of fear. Each time you are looking for somebody to blame, just check the mirror any person you see in there, just hold that person responsible. We begin to exhibit the mind-set of fear when we ignore our self concept and self esteem. On the other hand, behaviorists see fear from the learning perspective which is as a result of classical or instrumental conditioning. According to behaviorist it could also be the result of accidental pairing or wrong learning processes. In order words, we sometimes learn fear and in most cases, the thing we attached out minds to become source of our fear. Fear is also learnt through wrong association. You begin to fear when you connect with the wrong persons.

From the spiritual angle, fear is a natural phenomenon; fear came into existence when sin entered the world. God has continuously reminded us about fear and the solution to it.

For instant, in Genesis 32, Jacob became afraid of his brother Esau and prayed "Deliver me, I pray thee, from the hand of my brother, from the hand of Esau: **for I fear him**, lest he will come and smite me, and the mother with the children." In 1 Chronicles 28: 20; David was telling his son Solomon to be strong and of good courage and go on with the battle of life. He went on to remind him not to fear nor be dismay, for God will be with him in all he does. The same thing happened to Joshua in Joshua 1:5, when God reminded him not to fear but be of good courage. One thing I notice here is that each time the Bible mention fear, courage or strength will follow. Can you imagine David and Joshua, Gideon and many other God's heroes and leaders experiencing fear yet God was always there? The same thing will still be your portion if you put your faith and trust in God. You can still see the Bible for further reading on fear- Hebrews 13:5, 1 Chronicles 22:13, 1 Samuel 20:13. In facts, fear appears more than 365 times in the Bible, meaning there is fear in each day. It seems to be one word that has appeared more than many words in the Bible.

One thing we need to understand is that fear and faith are both contagious. We become infected with fear when we are surrounded with people infected by fear. We also become brave and courageous when we are surrounded by people with tangible faith solidly based on God's word. It is also noteworthy that you can as well infect others. It is a matter of who you connect with. It takes one man to infect a whole community with fear. It also takes one man to strengthen the unity of the entire community. In Judges 7:3-6, there were two set of people infected with fear (1) Those that were able to show or express their fears and (2) Those that hid their fear within their minds. When Gideon identified this problem, he said, whosoever is **fearful and afraid**, let him return and depart early from mount Gilead. And there returned of the people **twenty and two thousand**; and there remained **ten thousand**. While twenty two thousand that were able to express their fear left, out of ten thousand soldiers, nine thousand and seven hundred still pretended to be bold and courageous. Gideon saw ten thousand brave soldiers but God saw only three hundred soldiers. It was not the crowd but the contents of their minds. In Verse 4, God gave Gideon a test to prove his army, and God said the people are yet too many; bring them down unto the water, and **I will try them** for thee there: and it shall be, that of whom I say unto thee, This shall go with thee, the same shall go with thee; and of **whomsoever I say unto thee**, This shall not go with thee, the same shall not go. In the end of the day, there were only three hundred men. We should also guard against associating with losers or men with loose mind because they will unconsciously and consciously influence our actions in a negative way.

TWO TYPES OF FEAR

1. **THE FEAR OF GOD**: This type of fear has to do with reverence for God. It is unlike the abnormal fear of inexistence

fear of nothing. This type of fear is beneficiary and healthy to the mind, soul and body. It helps us guide our steps as we move through the echelon of life. It provides us a pathway to approach life in different dimension. Proverb 9:10 says, "A wise man start his journey of life with the fear of God. It is the type of fear that helps us expresses God' sovereignty and dignity in a unique way. This type of fear prompted David to say "..... Destroy him not: for **who can stretch forth his hand** against the LORD's anointed, and be guiltless? The LORD **forbids** that I should stretch forth mine hand against the LORD's anointed. This type of fear prompted the mid wives in Exodus 1:17 and 21 to saved baby Moses. This type of fear also helped Moses to appreciate the goodness of God's deliverance and faithfulness when Moses said who is like unto thee, O LORD, among the gods? Who is like thee, glorious in holiness, **fearful in praises**, doing wonders? This type of fear helped Brother Job hold on to God faithfulness when the Bible declared

"That Job was perfect and upright, and one that **feared God**, and eschewed evil." It is the same fear that favors us with God's grace. Psalm 33:18 says "behold, the eye of the LORD is upon them that **fear him**, upon them that hope in his mercy." Proverbs 1:7 says "The fear of the LORD is the beginning of knowledge: but fools despise wisdom and instruction." This type of fear equips us instead of destroying us. It prepares us for the future instead of taking us to the past. When the God kind of fear is in us, we become brave, focus and courageous.

2.   **THE DEVIL'S KIND OF FEAR:** This type of fear expresses the presence of evil forces in our minds. The fear that something evil is about to take place or befall us. The same Job that held God faithfully and fear him, suddenly manifested abnormal fear and the Bible said fear came upon me, and trembling, which made all my bones to shake. This indicates that fear is a spirit. The same father Israel that beheld God's fear when he wrestled the Holy Spirit and named

a place "**PENIEL**" suddenly allowed circumstances of life grip him. He prayed and said Lord "deliver me, I pray thee, from the hand of my brother, Esau: for I fear him, **lest he will come and smite me**, and the mother with the children." Jacob became afraid that his brother will kill. These situations are triggered when we begin to step out of God's circle. In most cases, we tend to look backward just like Brother Paul when he took his sight out of Jesus. Matthew 14:30 says "But when he saw the wind boisterous (He look at the challenge of life rather than Jesus), **he became afraid**; and **beginning to sink**. We become vulnerable to life threatening situations such as fear to die, fear to fail, fear to see or witness and the fear to experience when we take our focus from Jesus Christ. This type of fear happens when there is the absence of God's perfect love. We are afraid of people because we do not love and trust them. We are afraid that they might hurt us. Sometimes, we are even afraid of ourselves. We hate who we are, we want to be like the other person, do things other people do. We are afraid because we allow miserable situations over-shadow our minds. Jude 1:12 says, "These are spots in your feasts of charity, when they feast with you, **feeding themselves without fear**." But the only thing that conquers it all is God's love. I John 4:18 says, **"There is no fear** in love; but perfect love casteth out fear: because fear hath torment. He that feareth is not made perfect in love." A writer once said do not tell God how huge your storm is, tell the storm how gigantic your God is.

HOW DO WE LEARN FEAR

Until you tell yourself this bitter truth that the fear of suffering is worse than the suffering itself you will forever remain the worst victim of fear. There are various ways we learn fear. We learn to fear by classically conditioning our mind to some certain things.

We learn fear by incorporating pictures of things in our minds through negative reactions. Here is an example to show how this works... a girl who is afraid of insect

(Entomophobia) watch insect on the television react negatively. Present to her a toy insect time over time, you will notice that at a point her response to this stimulus become inbuilt (reflex). She may grow with this unconscious action overtime. At this point unconditional response has become part of her any time she sees a toy insect. She may show some signs of maturity and the ability to control her reacting impulse but the unconscious mannerism will always manifest itself. People attached their fear to a particular variable. To some, fears of image (Iconophobia), fear of learning (sophophobia), fear of fire (pyrophobia), fear of public places, crowds (agoraphobia), fear of water(hydrophobia) etc. In other words, these diseases are sometimes as a result of poor learning processes.

We also learn fear by incorporating our pagan cultural values into our daily lives. As Christians, it is our duty to transform lives positively but paganism has now become part of our Christian practices. We now dress, dance, and sing Christian-pagan-like dresses and songs in the church. Our modern days preaching have also taken the form of materialism. In Nigeria for instance, culture of superstition such fear of lizard, chameleon, spider, and other natural factors have also affected our Christian growth and development. Colossians 3:10, rightly said it, "And have put on the **new man**, which is renewed in knowledge after the image of him (Jesus Christ) that created him." Ephesians 4:22 said "that ye put off concerning the **former conversation the old man**, which is corrupt according to the deceitful lusts." Romans 6:6 put it this way, "Knowing this, that our **old man** (the pagan man) is crucified with him, that the body of sin might be destroyed, that henceforth we should not serve sin (fear)."

CAUSES OF FEAR

SIN: This implies deviating from God's moral and spiritual laws. God never created us with fear until sin entered us. The number one cause of fear is sin. When God created man, there was nothing like fear until man deviated from God's standard. Then fear entered man. That was the genesis of fear.

TEMPERAMENT: Temperamental disorder is a good source of abnormal fear. It is abnormally developed from the mind as a variable tool for survival. In most cases, it is attributed to genetic factors. A situation when fear becomes an inheritable trait.

CHILDHOOD NEGLECT: Our adulthood is determined by childhood upbringing. Childhood maltreatment, lack of care and love and other forms of child abuse may subject a child to develop distrust and doubt and pave way for abnormal fear.

INFERIORITY COMPLEX: This can be described as an unrealistic feeling of inadequacy of the self. It is characterized by lack of self worth, poor self concept, doubt and uncertainty. These types of people usually fail to measure up with psychological, social and spiritual standard. These override negative emotional feelings pave way to irrational fear about life.

ERRONEOUS BELIEFS: The fundamental idea here is that fear is caused by the things we say to ourselves about the world and about ourselves. The beliefs that some certain things exist that affect us. For instance, most people believe that seen a black cat in the morning is a bad omen. Others believes that seen a rabbit during day time could be a sign of death. In erroneous belief, we incorporate some erroneous cultural conviction into our day to day lifestyle.

POOR LEARNING PROCESSES: Learning is an essential tool of human attribute. A poor learning process is a product of abnormal perception which is embedded in the unconscious mind. Whatsoever we learn from our childhood to later stage of life, manifest itself consciously or unconsciously. If we learn the wrong way, we exhibit abnormal behaviors. The end result is usually associated with fear of the unknown.

SITUATION OF LIFE SUCH AS TRAUMA: One thing about trauma is flash back response. Fearful responses also appear to be hardwired in the brain. Everything we do fall back to our brain. Our mind is not only a processing and storage device but serve as an internal camera that automatically flash back stored events. These flash back memories are activated by pictures of present events such as birthdays, funerals, stories, internal reflection of the past. At times, Guilty feelings may serve as a trigger factor.

DANGERS ASSOCIATED WITH FEAR:

AT HOME: Fear can be such a dangerous weapon of disunity in the family. Fear does not only give way to distrust but tearing the house into different part mostly when the presence of God is ignored. Firstly, the negative outcome speaks majorly on children who are the most vulnerable and fragile persons in the house. This happen when such children are exposed to neglect, constant abuse, unfriendliness and aggressiveness. In most cases when parent quarrel and argue, the impact rest on the child who knows nothing about it. We should also note that children learn through observation. Poor communication between parents can be very dangerous. This is where parents begin to develop fear and distrust for each other. I am afraid if I tell him the way I feel. He may yell at me or he may not believe me. He may not listen to what I have to say. Mind you, the house is the basic institution for molding the true personality of any child. It is the way you dress your house that people outside address you and your family. Parents sometime fail to know this erroneous attitude. They are afraid that if they tell their children the truth, they will not love them anymore. Such beliefs are a misconception and lies from the bottom of hell. Tell your child the truth even in the face of pain. It is better to tell your child the truth that will lead to his blessing than keeping away the truth from him that will lead to his pains.

SCHOOL: It is just a pity to say that our schools which are supposed to be centered for learning and human transformation have performed below average mark. The danger associated with fear in school is that such students are usually afraid to speak publicly. They are afraid to express themselves openly. They are afraid that others might laugh them at the slightest mistake they make. This in turn affects learning process. These students may not be able to learn the right way because fear has become a predisposition factor in their minds hindering learning and learning process. They may be shying away from handling responsibilities assigned to them. A very dangerous instrument that has helped many students buries their potentials without knowing same.

WORKING PLACE: Each time I look at people who abscond from taken responsibilities, I do not see their inabilities to perform a particulars task effectively but see a prolong disorder that was incorporated into their unconscious being. That is how fear work. Fear is learnt and become part of the individual overtime. It is not that they cannot do it but that they are afraid that they might not do it well. Let me say one thing you do not know; nobody was born with skill, all skills are learnt just like fear is learnt. It is what you do that makes the different. Those with fear disorder usually displace it on others through aggressiveness and displaced anger.

CHURCH: I think this is where the major problem lies. This is because fear has hindered evangelism and people can no longer tell others about the truth (Jesus Christ) John 14:6. Many Christians are failing to take the advantage they have to proclaim or evangelize the gospel and even share their faith by leading others to Christ. The major problem here is that they are riddled with fear, fear that people will say something they never wish to ear. I think the major problem is the concentration of sermons on fund raising, blessings and miracles for sale rather than solving critical issues such as spiritual and psychological challenges affecting an average individual in our society. Our minds are riddles with materialistic sermons; gospel Christian music and messages have become monetized and commercialized.

SOCIAL CONTEXT: This has to do with forming social relationship with others. His thought and belief about others is based on the fact that he misinterprets mental information about himself and others around him. Sometimes, he feels he cannot cope with them, that is to say, he is inferior to them. Fear causes inferiority complex. Inferiority complex, according to Alfred Adler indicates such characteristics as shyness, cautions, pedantry, and failure to function effectively. It is rooted in the individual lacking self esteem, confidence and fear of critics. Here the individual manifest some personality disorders such as stage fright, social withdrawal, paranoid personality disorder (suspicious of others), avoidance personality disorder (avoiding others may be due to experienced rejection of the past) and many others. In whichever way, he is afraid to express his view.

REMEDY TO THE PROBLEM OF FEAR:

First and foremost love yourself and see others as if you are seeing yourself. Your self esteem is the trueness of who you are. This can only be possible if you step out of your comfort zone and spiritual limitation. Poverty is not a problem except that human beings do limit their mental power by consciously or unconsciously declaring that this is who they are. According to some of them, this is how they met the system, their forefathers were in this condition and that there is no need. This is how God wills it. Human beings are made to break out of poverty by first breaking the power of limitation surrounding them. As a matter of fact, poverty is a starting point for any great achiever. That is why you must step out of your comfort zone. You must love everything about you, what you do, how you do and you will know that there is something about you that no other person has. But when you allow the spirit of fear get hold of you, it will paralyze you and make you feel inferior for no just cause. When Joseph discovered this secret, he said unto them, Fear not: for am I in the place of God? (Genesis 50:19). When Moses realized that his people were gripped with fear he said "**Fear ye not**, standstill, and see the salvation of the LORD, which he will shew to you today: for the Egyptians (challenges) whom ye have seen today, ye shall see them again no more (overcome) forever" (Exodus 14:13). God once reminded Joshua, Be strong and of a good courage, **fear not**, nor be afraid of them: for the LORD thy God, he it is that doth go with thee; he will not fail thee, nor forsake thee, (Deuteronomy 31:6)

Let me tell you one thing about fear, you sometimes learn fear unconsciously (that is without knowing), just like you are learning to read and write. You fear that you will fail, or make mistakes. The good news is that if you learn a particular behavior or attitude, you can also unlearn that behavior. The only time when fear is learnt automatically is when you experienced an acute shock as in accident, or in sudden death you witness. Apart from that fear that involves a timely reinforcement can also be reserved through unlearn process (That is the reversing method).

The only moment you should exercise fear in your life is when you are in the presence of God. Ecclesiastes 12:13, says, **the end of the mater**; all has been heard **Fear God** and keep his commandment. The Proverbs says in chapter 1 verse 7, the fear of God is the beginning of wisdom, in Chapter 15 verse 33, and it says the fear of God is instruction in wisdom. In Psalm 115:33, it says blessed are those who fear God. The fear of God is not timidity but humility. The fear of God is not stupidity but wisdom (The fear of the LORD is the beginning of knowledge: but fools despise wisdom and instruction. Psalm 1:7)

Development of the self is another major aspect that overcomes fear. Each time you look at yourself and say some optimistic words with faith, you energize your inner being (Mind and soul). When you keep doing this overtime, you begin to reinforce your inner, your spirit. Each time you do this, the spirit of fear in you is replaced with the spirit of boldness. Have you ever had a deep thought of I Timothy 1:7 that God did not give you the spirit of timidity (fear) but a spirit of power and self control? Let me tell one secret about inferiority complex, you have so much (potentials) to give that you do not know which one to fully maximize. So you are confused on which one to give. That is fear for you.

HUMAN HEALTH: People tend to ignore the potential dangers associated with fear in relation to human health. Have you ever noticed how your heart beats when you noticed something dangerous or threatening? If you look carefully, you will also notice that your eyes suddenly become red. More so, your skin become cool, your lips also become dry, you notice your heart pumping more than the normal way you should breathe. I think these are the visible signs you noticed when you exhibit fear. Are you also aware that irrational fear also paralyses mental activities, disrupt digestive functioning, disrupt kidney function and other physiological process you are not even aware of. The other negative effective effect of unnecessary fear is that it leads to rise in blood pressure, kidney malfunctioning and other physiological processes. Tim and Beverly Lahaye (1995) in their research also discovered that fear also causes strokes, goiter, diabetes, arthritis, headaches. Psychologically, fear causes emotional disturbances and confusion. Spiritually, it deprives us from communicating effectively with God during prayer. It makes us spiritually sick. It makes us lack internal peace. It also affects our relationship with others.

Apart from spiritual dangers associated with fear, some aspect of fearful responses appear to be hardwired in the brain and do not require learning (Seely, Stephen and Tate- 2008). When fear becomes a constant behavior, it evokes some abnormal response in the cerebral cortex. That gives reason some people manifest some abnormal psychological reflexes even when there is no just cause for such reflex action.

Sometimes, we learn how to fear unconsciously but we can still unlearn fear consciously. The truth of the matter is there are no magic drugs to fight back fear except through the following steps (a) You must first discover and accept fear as a problem (b) You must go for the root cause (c) Ask yourself why do you feel that way and act the way you do. Certain questions must be asked and answered.

It is foolish to fear what is not seen. What distinguish between losers and winners are the pictures they develop in their minds. When you develop negative pictures, you fear things that do not exist. It is what you see in your mind that attracts what comes to you. You first see the things of life inside your mind before they manifest on the outside.

CHAPTER 5
DOUBT

one thing I discovered in my state of persistent state of doubt was that each atom of doubt pushed me to faith.

When I was growing up, my greatest problem was not fear, anxiety, pride, nor the act of unforgiveness but the deep and chronic state of doubt. I almost doubted everything about myself. I almost doubted the power of miracle. I doubted the power of positivity. So I almost became a pessimist. My friends will always remind me of my potentials but I ignored or took for granted what they were saying. The power of doubt can be frustrating and challenging mostly when you are outside God's premises. Doubt can sometime pushed us to do the unexpected and imaginable mostly when are in an impossible position. But one thing I discovered in my state of persistent state of doubt was that each atom of doubt pushed me to faith. At a point, I discovered that those things I doubted myself were the things that brought me joy of the mind. Those things I doubted myself of, were the things I was doing better than ever expected. For instance, when I was in my junior secondary school, my History teacher will asked me to teach the junior ones and I will shy away in my frustration. I will always say I cannot do it. My social study teacher also saw this gift in me and gave me the same task and I will give the same excuse. So I was avoiding these two teachers who discovered who I was and my possibility of being a future teacher. But sometimes unconsciously, I will be teaching without knowing I was doing it. In my higher institution, the same thing happens and I shy away. The bottom line is that **doubt can only keep you away for a while but will never stop you from who you are**. I came to discovered that **the genesis for every hero begins with doubt**. Doubt serves as a stepping stone for faith. Every great man will always ask himself these simple yet a thousand and one questions, **"Can I do it?", "Is it possible?" "Is there any way out?"** These three questions are just the reverse order of "I can do it", "It is possible", and "there is a way out".

If you think there is no pride in you, there is no persistence and irrational fear in you, perhaps, doubt is another weakness or put it another plague that has cripple many great men and their spirituality mostly the righteous ones. Let's take a look at what doubt caused to many men of God. Doubt is so powerful that at any instance it can demolish a whole mountain of faith. It can take you one thousand years to build faith but doubt will erode it in just one minute. It takes doubt to welcome fear and anxiety into any man. Peter did not experience fear immediately; it was doubt the opposite of faith that attracted fear before he started sinking. In Luke 1:13-18 Zechariah did not only fear but doubted God's words **"how shall I know this?"** evidence of doubt, **"for**

I am an old man", behold he paid for it. All his righteousness did not count; he became deaf and dumb for a season till the wife put to birth. Doubt contradicts the sovereignty of God, his promises and blessings for us. Each time you doubt you make God a liar. The truth is this, when God is push out of a person life, doubt sets in and quickly build a debilitating fear- The Good News Magazine (2009).

Any victim of doubt is a pessimist, he lacks faith, and such person is filled with the spirit of unbelief. He rarely sees anything good out of anything. He is the type that will always refuse to rise up. They are the type that will always say can anything good come out of Israel? The good news is that in a trouble world full of sad news, there are bound to be men who will always say God is God, and we will never give up. Those who doubt themselves usually hate themselves and when you hate yourself, hardly will you appreciate anything you do. One thing about doubt is that it can help focus on the past but faith helps us to see a bright and beautiful future. The only thing I know is that there is a kind of doubt that triggers God to prove Himself beyond our imagination. When Gideon asked for a sign was because he doubt if God's hand was still in the affair of Israelites. Doubt became the only instrument to trigger God to prove himself. When God say "I am who I am", to many the statement is more or less hypothetic or abstract. God then will act on their state of doubt to prove Himself a faithful God.

Denis Waitley once said "if you believe you can, you probably can. If you believe you won't, you most assuredly won't. Belief is the ignition switch that gets you off the launching pad." Belief and doubt are both ignition switches that determine the road map your destiny. Those whose mind are led or configured by doubt will have their mind narrow down to pessimism while those whose mind are programmed by faith based on the word of positivity become optimists. At this point, it is not what we see with our eyes but what our minds see in the future. The human mind is a unique kingdom of its own, perfectly designed to direct the path of the future. It takes doubt to mar the brightness and glorious treasures of the future and also take faith to design the way to that glorious city. The reality here is that faith and doubt have remained two rivals in the mind of an average person. The power to determine who rule and take possession lies on the individual.

Charles Hummel asserts that, "A stronger faith can emerge through a siege of doubt; both holiness and faith are forged in the fires of temptation. Virtually every observer agrees that not only faith, but Christian growth and greater certainty, conviction, and service can result (and often does) from successfully dealing with one's uncertainty.

It is also important to note that both in the Old and New Testaments great miracles and heroes started with doubt. Gideon first doubted God after experiencing many challenges. He doubted the glory of God during his era, to him, if the presence and grace of God was with his father and great grand fathers. In some instances the complaints against God come into sight out of the ordinary and astonishingly strong. The name Isaac came as a result of doubt. Genesis 17:17 said "then Abraham fell upon his face, and laughed, and **said in his heart, Shall a child be born unto** him that is an hundred years old? and shall Sarah, that is ninety years old, bear? Sarah laughter brought the name Isaac because of doubt of possibility.

Job almost fall prey of doubt when faced with trial and tribulations, his encounter with the Lord brought about the resolution of his doubts, repentance and trust in God, leading to his multiple blessings (Job 42). This prompted Job to make one of the most remarkable statements in the Bible, "I **know my redeemer liveth**". The Psalmist expressed doubt, but it became an avenue to express positive attitude of praise to God (Ps. 42:5-6, 11; 43:5).

Doubt sometimes helps us to develop a unique attitude of retracing our missing steps. We can never miss our ways and remain there. Faith can never just come up all of a sudden. It must start with an atom of doubt.

LET'S LOOK AT SOME HEROES OF DOUBT

1. Abraham, when God told him he would be a father in old age. "Then Abraham fell upon his face, and **laughed**, and **said in his heart**, Shall a child be born unto him that is an hundred years old? and shall Sarah, that is ninety years old, bear?" (Genesis 17:17)

2. When Sarah heard she would be a mother in her old age. She **laughed within herself**, saying, after I am waxed old shall I have pleasure, **my lord being old also**? (Genesis 18:12).

3. Moses, when God asked him to lead the children of Israel out of Egypt to the Promised Land. He gave two excuses because of doubt (Exodus 14:1 and 10), And Moses answered and said, but, behold, **they will not believe me**, nor hearken unto my voice: for they will say,

the LORD hath not appeared unto thee. And Moses said unto the LORD, Oh my LORD, **I am not eloquent**, neither heretofore, nor since thou hast spoken unto thy servant: but **I am slow of speech**, and **of a slow tongue**.

4. Gideon when God appointed him a judge and leader (Judges 6:14-23). He doubted God's presence during his time and even said, Oh my Lord, if the LORD be with us, why then is all this befallen us? Where be all his miracles which our fathers told us of, saying, Did not the LORD bring us up from Egypt? But now the LORD hath forsaken us, and delivered us into the hands of the Midianites. He even requested God' sign and miracle.

5. The Bible said Zechariah prayed and his prayer was heard, (Luke 1:13) but he doubted his ability to father a child. In verse 20, the Angel of the Lord told him you will be mute and not be able to speak until the day these things take place. In Luke 1:13-18 Zechariah did not

only fear but doubted God's words "**how shall I know this?" evidence of doubt, "for I am old man"**.

6. John the Baptist was a typical example of doubt, when he asked, is this the Jesus Christ (the Messiah) or are we expecting? It is presumed that he was triumphant over his doubt, for in spite of it (and even during it!) Jesus pronounced his great compliment about John (Matt. 11:11; Luke. 7:28). (Jn. 20:28).

7. Thomas more far-reaching doubt, in spite of Jesus' rebuke, led to Thomas glorious recognition of Jesus' divinity, I think I should describe this man as the father of doubt. His level of doubt was so pronounced, throughout his discipleship with Jesus Christ, he never changed. I still can find out why (John 20:24,25).

In Matthew 21:21, Jesus once said unto them, Verily I say unto you, If ye **have faith, and doubt not**, ye shall not only do this which is done to the fig tree, but also if ye shall say unto this mountain,

Be thou removed, and be thou cast into the sea; it shall be done.

One remarkable thing about these set of people is that God used them to accomplish great signs and wonders in the Bible. God prove to them great patience because he understood their minds. A writer wrote, **"Honest Doubt was not a bad starting point as long as they did not stay there."** – Author Unknown.

THE DANGERS ASSOCIATED WITH DOUBT

1.   Doubt neutralizes faith. It weakens faith. Doubt is the opposite and antagonist of faith. Each time you allow the spirit of doubt enter you, you automatically pursue faith out of you.

2.   Doubt makes us lose concentration. Each time you doubt, you will be having many thoughts. In most cases, there is intra-psychic conflict of decision making. Sometime, we may doubt subject to doubt ourselves, between the word of God and Satan?

3.   During doubting we exhibit some level of psychological discomfort such as confusion, uncertainty, worry and even fear of nothing. This is because we are at a cross road thinking which way to go.

I Timothy 2:8, "I will therefore that men pray everywhere, lifting up holy hands, without wrath and doubting".

HOWEVER, THE FOLLOWING COULD BE HELPFUL:

Doubt is an evidence of absolute lack of the knowledge of God not minding the situation. Believe is a product of the mind, create that picture in your mind that God exist and that his promises are true. The most successful men are those that make God's promises their foundation and back up. All things worketh together for good to those that believe means every circumstances that generate doubt, anger, fear and anxiety are designed to catapult you to your next level in life. Great men don't just wake over night to their thrones, no; hurdles and trials are defined as stepping stones. All you need is to develop faith, make it an instrument of survival. Greatness is not the product of what your face look like but the function of the mindset. Greatness is also not by chance but the configuration of the mindset.

Greatness is the product of the mind that reflects in the physical appearance of a man. Faith is the opposite of doubt and unbelief, faith is always on the other side of the river while doubt and unbelief the other side. The secret is just ability to configure your mindset to see the goodness of life, level of courage, determination and ability to speak positivity into your life to make the desire change.

Do not be short sighted, for the future to be better, it only depends on your mental perception and spiritual development. Faith is all about mentality for self empowerment, mentality to extraordinary and divine empowerment. For out of great imagination come a better and bright future, a realistic tomorrow and a financial fulfillment in life. It all starts with the walls of your mind.

CHAPTER 6
ANGER

Moses was so angered that what he suffered for forty days and night got smash up within a twinkle of an eye.

Many people seem to have the notion that anger is sometime a justifiable trait. To them anger is natural, so every man gets angry. Anger seems to be a man's way of expressing his frustration and internal conflict. But then many have refused to acknowledge the fact that anger is a temporary state of insanity. Anger is a destroyer. Anger follows hostility and aggressiveness and leads to our inabilities to control sound judgment and thinking. Anger is not only a psychosocial problems but a spiritual cankerworm. I do not neglect the bible saying be angry but sin not (Ephesians 4:26). The Bible does not tell us that we should not feel angry, but in a way not to allow anger subjects us to sin. **We can never avoid been angry but we can control those things that make us angry.** We can as well program our minds to absorb the way we react to anger.

It also pointed out that it is very important to control our anger in a way that will not hurt our emotions. Paul reminded us that if we bottled up anger inside of us, it can cause us to remain bitter and destroy from within. Anger is a time bomb in our mind but it is triggered by external factors such as events of frustration, inability to achieve a target, failures, friends and relatives. Here we might destroy our relationship with others as well as depriving the Holy Spirit to have a place in our mind. The wisest man had this warning for us, **"a stone is heavy, and the sand weighty; but a fool's wrath is heavier than them both."** He went further to express the degree of anger by saying "wrath is cruel, and anger is outrageous." (Proverbs 27:4).

Happiness, fear, anger, sadness and disgust are five emotions most often regarded as being basic to all humans- Robert Sternberg (2001). It can be seen as a feeling of frustration or inability to achieve a specify goal. Most of the time, we direct anger toward others, people we love, if they fail us. In most cases, we direct it inwardly, when we measure ourselves below average. The dangers associated with anger in recent research indicate that most of man's ill health are related to anger, interpersonal conflict and inability to solve problems the right way. Anger, hostility, wrath, malice….. as the Bible calls it, is enmity against our souls. Anger does not only destroy home, friendship, health but life.

Proverb 14:7, "He that is soon angry dealeth foolishly: and a man of wicked devices is hated."

21:19, "It is better to dwell in the wilderness, than with a contentious and an angry woman."

22:24, "Make no friendship with an angry man; and with a furious man thou shalt not go."

25:23, "The north wind driveth away rain: so doth an angry countenance a backbiting tongue."

Ecclesiastes 7:9, "Be not hasty in thy spirit to be angry: for anger resteth in the bosom of fools."

It is obvious to say that even though anger is universally seen as a natural phenomenon, it is *destructive*, though not all anger is sin. Temporal reaction to actions or events may not be seen as sin, but when it persists beyond the ordinary measure, it becomes sin. If God is slow to anger (Nahum 1:3) yet remain supreme in majesty and power, then who are you to be quick in anger? The best way to justify anger could best be seen in Ephesians 4:26-27 which states: **in your *anger* do not *sin*;** do not let the sun goes down while you are still *angry*, and do not give the devil a foothold (NIV).

Though we should not take for granted and abuse the above Bible portion, as many may say. It is very dangerous whether five second or more, do not give room to anger. It can become part of you and occupy your spiritual entity.

Consider these Bible verses carefully.

1. Be not hasty in thy spirit to be angry; for anger resteth in the bosom of fools. (Ecclesiates 7:9)
2. Cease from anger, and forsake wrath. (Psalm 37:8)
3. Make no friendship with an angry man; and with a furious man thou shall not let go: Lest thou learn his ways and get snare to thy soul. (Proverbs 22:24
4. Better is a dry morsel and quietness therewith, than a house full of sacrifices with strife. (Proverbs 17:1)
5. It is better to dwell in the wilderness than with a contentious and an angry woman (Proverbs 15:18)

6. Hatred stirred up strife: but love covers all sins (Proverbs 10:12).
7. Wherefore, my beloved brethren, let every man be swift to hear, slow to speak, slow to wrath: for the wrath of man worketh not the righteousness of God. (James 1:19-20).
8. But now put away all these; **anger**, strife, malice, blasphemy, filthy communication out of your mouth. (Colossian 3:8)

The only way out to control anger, strife, hostility and the rest of them all, is to keep away from all form of bitterness, anger, malicious thoughts, wrath and evil speaking. Keep away from stimulating provoking items such as aggressive movies, pictures and evil-friends. All these have a significant impact in our lives. Therefore, learn to practice kindness, love, charity, tenderhearted, forgiveness, giving, hospitality (Ephesians 4:31-32, if there any virtue, praise, think on these things, Philippians 4:8). Learn how to smile and be happy all the time; the truth is that happiness and joy gives you life and make you younger but what anger takes from you cannot be restored in just an hour. That is the reason each time you are angered, you hardly recover within a short time.

LEVEL AT WHICH ANGER MANIFEST ITSELF

The first level of anger includes the introduction phase. At this phase, a stimulus is introduced to elicit a particular physiological reaction. For instance, a man is faced with a situation that may make him annoy. In this phase, it is easy to identify the problem mostly when we can exhibit humility.

The arousal phase is next and can be disastrous if care is not taken, unlike the introductory phase where we can identify the source of the problem. The arousal phase follows an abnormal reaction and arousal of the physiological functioning. This includes abnormal secretion of the neurotransmitters, high blood pressure, redness of the eyes, dryness of the mouth, and many other abnormal brain processes. This phase is relatively very short and can be disastrous. This is the destructive phase when action is exhibited. The time frame here is short and quick.

The third is the **resolution phase**, it is the regretful stage. In Exodus 32:19. 28:24. 12:18, we saw the damage caused by Moses' state of anger. He was so angered that what he suffered for forty days and night, got smash up within a twinkle of an eye. The Tablet containing the Ten Commandments was not only broken but resulted to the death of about three thousand men. In the resolution phase, we try to repair the damage and of course we know how costly it used to be. In this phase, a whole lot of people usually make this regretful silly comment; "had I know", "I did not know it will happen this way", "oh my God......" and many other remorseful statements.

The summary of this message is this; guide against phase one and you will not see yourself in the resolution phase trying to amend what you labor for, the long relation you establish with people around you, even God and the Holy Spirit.

SIGNS/CHARACTERISTICS THAT SHOWS ANGER

1. A feeling of tension
2. Stress reaction and aggression
3. Reaction formation
4. Displacement of emotional feelings
5. Psychological discomfort
6. Redness of the eyes
7. Abnormal sweating
8. Increase bodily temperature
9. Temporary Cognitive imbalance

HOW CAN YOU CONQUER ANGER

Acknowledging that there is a problem is the ultimate. Then followed by personal change of decision is the next number key to anger management. If you are a new man like the one described in Ephesians 4:21-24 "indeed you have heard him (Jesus)..... that you put off your former conduct (anger) the old man which grow corrupt and put on the new man (holiness in Christ). In other word, **you can change thing and get control** of your anger.

In Psychology, according to social learning theory, behavior is learnt and still can be unlearnt. Most of our bad actions form our behaviors. The truth is, we can still unlearn them by replacing them with good ones. This can be done by **(a) Meditating on the word** of God on daily basis (Joshua 1:6-7), **(b)** feeding our minds with the right foods Philippians 4:9 "The things which you **learned** and received and heard and saw in me, these do, and the peace of God will be with you.

Happiness and joy are two ingredients you can never find in another man's garden of life. What I mean is this; nobody will give you these two things the way you give to yourself. Nobody will give you happiness and joy if you do not first give it to yourself. It is not found in food, drink, or anything outside your mind. Anger can only be control when you are able to control the state of your mind. We are to be gentle to ourselves, humble fair-minded and charitable to those outside the church.

Consistence spiritual exercise will help you grow in faith and character. It is what we do that attracts others to see the radiating power of the Holy Spirit in us. Those who practice consistence spiritual exercise of the mind do not talk much, they do not quarrel, they are not easily angered, and they do not easily react to physical challenges or temptations.

FOOD FOR THOUGHS

The monsters of the mind are far worse than those that actually exist. Fear, doubt, and hate have hamstrung more people than beasts ever have.
CHRISTOPHER PAOLINI,

Just as dogs love to chew bones, the mind loves to get its teeth into problems. That's why it does crossword puzzles and builds atom bombs.

ECKHART TOLLE, The Power of Now

The country would be far better if the population were half as interested in keeping their minds in as good condition as they tried to keep their bodies. **JOHN SAUL, Black Lightning.**

CHAPTER 7
ENVY/ JEALOUSY

When you feel you wish to be like the other person, you only deny or reject or even empty yourself of who you are by telling God he made mistake creating you the way you are.

In this chapter, I am going to combine two diseases because of their closeness in meaning. Though, many sees these two disease as singular as they are sometime used interchangeably. For instance, the English dictionary New Edition defines Jealousy as feeling of angry or unhappy because somebody you like or love is showing interest in somebody else. It could also be define as the feeling that you had something that someone else has. Envy on the other, envy is defined as the feeling of wanting to be in the same situation as somebody else. Envy and jealousy are two concepts we must guide against because in most cases, we feel we are doing the right thing. The writer of Proverbs had this to say wrath is cruel, and anger is outrageous; but **who is able to stand before envy**? One thing I have not earlier mentioned is that all these diseases discussed in this book are all fought within the mind. Though, they are fought in the mind of the individual but its consequences are spread in the lives of others. You should be mindful that anything you do affects the lives of others not just yourself.

When you smile at others they smile back at you except an average sadist. Envy is a twin brother of jealousy. It must not be allowed to grow root in our conscious, subconscious and super-conscious mind. Envy develops root and spread it branches in the lives of others. If it is not control on time, it gives way to bitterness. Bitterness gives way to hatred and hatred pave way to murder. The Bible rightly said it, he who **hate, envy, jealous or keep grudge inside him, the same is a murder and a murder has no place in**

God's place or put it eternal life (I John 3:15). Those who exhibit the spirit of envy and jealousy have venom of bitterness running in their veins.

The mind commands the body and immediately it obeys. The mind orders itself, and meets resistance.

BRIAN HERBERT & KEVIN J. ANDERSON, The Butlerian Jihad

Envy and Jealousy are silent barriers found in our houses, offices, schools and mostly inside God's house. No wonder you see many believers inside God's house for decades without any changes. Year in years out, their spiritual growth is still the same, no fruit to show, no personal change despite powerful message from powerful men of God. Envy/Jealousy paves way to hatred and bitterness. The conflict between Saul and David was nothing other than Envy and Jealousy which resulted to hatred. Saul refused to acknowledge that God blessed him differently from David. David had a unique gift which can never be compare to Saul's gift. Both of them had something different from each other. But Saul refused to acknowledge who he was, and the treasure inside of him. Let me tell you one thing here, each time you Envy and Jealous somebody simply because he did something spectacular, you will not only cause yourself heart attack but sudden and unnatural death will visit you. You should know that you are unknowingly telling God that he did not create you well.

Each time you exhibit any form of Envy and Jealousy, you begin to hate, then you allow spirit of bitterness to come in. bitterness and hatred are all silent killers. Envy and jealousy stir bitterness. Bitterness on the other hand can never make you better. They make the individual refuse to acknowledge who he is and what he can do. For any individual to be more pessimistic and less confident just allow Envy and Jealousy come into you. Look at what Envy and Jealousy does to the individual, it shrink your facial nerves and make you older and ugly. Envy and Jealousy only characterize your level of immaturity and spiritual deficiency in God.

Victims of Envy and Jealousy hardly smile; they hardly see anything good in themselves not even in others. Please just avoid it with prayers and fasting, give yourself joy, and make yourself happy, keeping your mind on the positive spiritual things is the only way out. See Proverb 6:34, "for Envy and Jealousy is the rage of a man, therefore he will not spare in the day of vengeance. Those with Envy and Jealousy syndrome are those who are fond of complaining in the church, work, family and school. These set of person are usually sadists. They will never appreciate any success.

Let me tell you something, you can never be sister "A," she may not say a word but the whole word will be shaking yet you may be so eloquent, your eloquences may not wave a death leave. So guide against it. Every human being is unique and gifted personally. No two persons have the same gift and talent. When you feel you wish to be like the other person, you only deny or reject or even empty yourself of who you are by telling God he made mistake creating you the way you are. Avoid statement such as I wish I was like Sis. Mary, Bro. Daniel rather appreciates what they have and who you are. Learn to focus on your strength, gift and talents- II Corinthians 8:12 "for if there be first a willing mind, it is accepted according to that a man hath, and not according to that he hath not.

CONSEQUENCES OF ENVY AND JEALOUSY

1) Envy and Jealousy are spiritual **jinx**, evil and a moral danger to humanity. They do not only affect our psychological and physiological state of mind but paralyses our spirituality.

2) Envy and Jealousy are pollutant to our minds. They bare our mind from seeing and hearing the word of God. Matthew 5:8 says they that worship him (God) must worship in him truth and purity and that only the pure in heart can see God.

How then can we worship him when our minds are filled with obnoxious substances and burdens that are inimical to God's provisions?

3) It creates room inside our minds to backbite others. Back biting is one thing that brought God's judgment against the children of Israel while in the wilderness.

4) It creates room for negative ideology and distorted picture about innocent people. The irony about Envy and Jealousy is that those people we envy may not know about it.

Sometimes, these people relate with us freely with open minds, while we are dying inside of us. We only feel the pains and distress alone and when we can no longer bear it, we resort to more deadly means of discharging our emotional conflict. That is what happened to Cain and Abel in the Bible, **why should God approved Abel's gift and not me?** So Cain devised a mean to discharge his emotional conflict. His Envy and Jealousy gave way to aggression and aggression led to the murder of Abel.

Envy and Jealousy are communicable disease. It attracts like-mind persons. This is because it starts from one person and spread to people of like minds. People hardly notice why a church will suddenly collapse. Envy and Jealousy are nurtured by one man and planted in the minds of others without knowing same. The devil is astute and smart; you **must** not neglect this fact. Why always brother "A"? is there no other person in the Church? This is a sign of the manifestation of Envy and Jealousy. The victim may not identify it. Please guide against it seriously. With envy and jealousy, we tend to focus on others and neglecting our talents. We feel we cannot what they can do but we also forget to realize that they cannot do what we can do.

Envy and Jealousy are psychological characteristics of inferiority complex. The simple truth about envy is that you can hardly confront the person and express your mind on how you feel about a particular situation. You suffer it more than the person you are looking at.

Envy and Jealousy do not give you the room to see good things in others. Even when they are doing good, or say the right thing we still not like what come out of them. Anything about them does not necessarily make any meaning to us.

One other funny thing about Envy and Jealousy is that it blinds and empties ourselves not to see our potentials. We only see ourselves from a wrong perspective. Every human being is a potential creature (Isaiah 43:7- "Everyone **who is called by my name, everyone whom I have created, whom I have formed for my Glory"**. In Psalm 100:3 it says "It is he (God) not we who made ourselves," You must acknowledge that fact. Then you must acknowledge your uniqueness (Personal talent or Gift) **Romans 12:6, " having then gifts differing according to the grace"** in our ways but Divinely connected in such a way that our potentials can only come to the light by what others do to us and what we do to them. Some people are somewhere to fulfill our divine assignment from the wrong perspective whiles others positively. Which one do you want to fulfill?

CHAPTER 8
UNFORGIVENESS

If you find yourself holding onto a grudge against someone who's grievously harmed you, for you to find a way to forgive them—for you to *become* the kind of person who *can*- just say these three words- " **I forgive you**"

The question will naturally come: why is it that some people cannot forgive, is it that they do not want to forgive or the memory of the past is always there? Is it about parents who have abused us, maltreated and/or subjected us to unbearable pains? This is because I have heard some youngsters saying, over my dead body will I forgive this woman/man so called my mother/father. In fact, one young lady while in police detention once told me I do not have a mother in the presence of her mother. What a pity. Is it about our children who have rebelled against us? Is it about our spouses who have abandoned, maltreated and/or subjected us to unbearable conditions? Should I mention friends who have betrayed us? Strangers who have treated us badly, misinterpret our hospitalities, harmed us or even killed our loved ones? Or even tyrants who have killed our families? Is Boko Haram, for example, not forgivable? Is it true that we can forgive somebody without forgiving what they did to us or our loved ones? Often time we forgive people without forgiving what they did to us or our loved ones. What then is forgiveness?

In most cases, we feel bad and sometime refuse to let go our past anger because we feel somebody has done us so much wrong and will not forgive them. In most times, we believe those who have offended us does not deserve our forgiveness, but that is not true. We can still forgive and live happily with each other. Some feel even if they forgive, the past will not be forgiven and forgotten. Here comes the question, who are you forgiving?

Is it the person, his action or both of them or yourself? We often time, feel those hurt took something from us, but the only thing that get back to us is forgivingness. When you refused to forgive people, you give power over you, you cage your mind and become psychological slave. When you forgive people without forgiven what they did to you, you leave debris of what they did to you in your mind. It is like sweeping a house half way. When you express total forgiveness, you get total control over them. You push over state of guilt back to them.

Few benefits of forgiveness
1. It increases man's self worth and confidence.
2. It enhances our spiritual state of mind.
3. It increases sense of self safety and security.
4. It increases our sense of happiness and joy. It empties our mind of spiritual or psychological debris.

The ability to forgive lies in the discovery of the curative nature of the power of forgiveness. It enables us to allow into our conception the possibility that they have positive characteristics or have the capability to do well and that we can still give them the second chance to improve.

Each time you forgive you do three things:

(1) You liberate your soul from condemnation. You are doom for condemnation because you have a burden and a picture of hatred of that person in your mind. That is why each time you see that person; you first get hurt by changing all physiological and psychological function of you.

(2) You liberate that person or persons from your mind. The truth is when you refused to forgive; you invariably tie that person(s) inside your mind. Your mind becomes a cage or prison to their happiness and freedom. That is why when they see you; they become angry and unhappy with themselves. Some wish they never see you. Your inability to

forgive other offends or even hurt them the more. You make them fear you the more.

(3) The major aspect of forgivingness lies in it curative nature of healing both of you. Forgiveness also helps us place our trust in other people's mind without fear, doubt, remorse or regret. Forgiveness therefore brings healing.

One secret to exercise the power of forgiveness lies in our ability to free ourselves. Self liberation is the state of mind fill with faith, peace, humility, prayer and love and devoid of hatred, grudges and apathy. Lack of forgiveness is an evil spirit and cannot dwell where there is happiness and joy. Happy is the man who walks in the way or in the integrity of God; his ways are upright and never walk in the integrity or the counsel of the wicked. One thing about unforgiving spirit is that it makes us more pessimistic and less optimistic, suspicious and lack trust in others even ourselves.

Therefore, learn to keep your mind on those things that are pure, moral, just, and holy, excellence, lovely. In fact, anything worthy of praise and adoration to the Almighty God is what is required of us by been a forgiver. By so doing, you program your mindset to be happy at all time. Each time you are happy you recreate and refresh your body system but when you are sad, unhappy, moody and pessimistic you destroy more than one thousand body cells for every minute. Imagine how many brain cells you destroy for just sixty minutes.

You need to acknowledge God through Jesus Christ in all you do, your health, your career, education, family, and anything you can ever mention. Galatians 4:7-8, put it this way, therefore you are no longer a slave (a slave to unforgiving spirit) but a son and an heir of God through Christ. In verse 8, it says but then, indeed, when you did not know God, you serve those things which by nature are gods, anything you put your trust outside God is your idol or gods. Those things continue to live within your mind. When you hold on to unforgiveness, you become a slave to the spirit of unforgiveness.

I would suggest this: If you find yourself holding onto a grudge against someone who has grievously harmed you, for you to find a way to forgive them—for you to *become* the kind of person who *can* and have the power to transform the life of the person you are forgiving, just say these three words- " **I forgive you**". It is not of course that easy but sometimes it remains the only and the best option in forgiving them. Then you are not only setting yourself free, you are actually contributing to something of greater importance in the live of that person. Something the world is factually crying out for in more places than you could in all probability imagine.

FACT ABOUT FORGIVENESS:

1. There is true freedom in absolute forgiveness.
2. Identify the reason for forgiveness.
3. The lack of forgiveness creates a prison in our minds where people are spiritually prisoned.

4. True forgiveness lies in the forgiveness of the self.
5. The prodigal son was forgiven long ago before he came to the father for forgiveness
6. The only quality that distinguished Nelson Mandela was his ability to forgive those who imprisoned him for twenty seven years.
7. The greatest forgiver is God. While we were yet sinner, he provided a perfect lamb for the remission of sin.
8. True forgiveness lies in the absolute release of the past evil from your mind, preparing your mind for the future and stepping into the future without bitterness, grudges and malice.
9. True forgiveness cure prolong hatred.
10. True forgiveness is a liberation weapon to Divine breakthrough.
11. There is no struggle in true forgiveness.
12. When you forgive, you forgive and let it go and never recall that picture in your mind again.

CHAPTER 9
PRIDE

One danger about pride is that it blinds the victim before his destruction, leading us to pomposity.

Pride can be defined as an unconscious effort for self glorification, or you can still define pride as any selfish action designed to attribute success to the self rather than God. Pride inflates the ego (our minds) and subjects the soul to some sort of pseudo confident and boldness. In most cases, it is misunderstood as the case may be with confidence. Pride inflates our ego; leading us to pomposity. Pride forces us to disobey and compare ourselves with people who are higher than us, thereby leading to unhealthy contention (Proverbs 13:10). Pride is a dangerous weapon for self destruction. We must guide against it if we want to attain that level of success and spiritual growth we deserved. Though, sometimes, taking joy in one's work or accomplishment in some works could be a healthy form of pride. To say that one is happy with an achieved goal by making statement such as; "Yes, I did it", " I won it" and many others could be a healthy pride, but when the glory and honor is not directed to the right direction or source to acknowledge God, it become sin. See what Apostle Paul had to say about self attribute (Pride) in the book of II Corinthians 10:2,12-16, " but I beseech you, that I may not be bold when I am present with that confidence, wherewith I think to be bold against some, **which think of us as if we walk according to the flesh**...... in verse 12, it reads, for we dare not make ourselves of the number, or compare ourselves with some that **commend themselves** (Pride); but they **measuring themselves by themselves** (self attribute, a characteristic of pride) and comparing themselves among themselves, are not wise........ in verse 15, reads, not boasting of things without our measure ...... of other men's work, but having hope, when your faith is increased.

ANGLES OF PRIDE: Pride is a spiritual virus. It is the number one diseases of kings and Rulers. If you have any cause to doubt ask mighty rulers like Shaka the Zulu, King Asa, King Joash, King Hezekiah, King Nebuchadnezzar and many others. Take a good study of Kings in the Bible; they had no other key challenge except pride. This has been the source to their fall. God said I will **break the pride of your power**; and I will make your heaven as iron, and your earth as brass- Leviticus 26:19. A man's pride shall bring him low: but honor shall uphold the humble in spirit.

SPIRITUAL POINT OF VIEW

Pride destroyed king Nebuchadnezzar, in the book of Daniel 4:30 "because the king said to himself, **is not this great Babylon which I have built with my OWN might power**..." while he was talking, the result came instantly. He attributed success to himself neglecting the presence and the might of God. The king did not only personalize himself but competed with God, trying to share in God's glory and honor. God is the only person that can use the first person pronoun "**I**" authoritatively, see for yourself in the book of Isaiah 43:10-11; 45:18,21-22, and 46:9-10. One danger about pride is that it blinds the victim before his destruction. It causes us to disobey. It leads us to commit sin without knowing that we are actually committing sin.

➢ **VICTIMS OF PRIDE IN THE BIBLE**

King Nebuchadnezzar   Daniel 4:37 and 5:20, "Now I Nebuchadnezzar praise and extol and honour the King of heaven, all whose works are truth, and his ways judgment: and those that walk in pride he is able to abase. But when his heart was lifted up, and his mind hardened in pride, he was deposed from his kingly throne, and they took his glory from him."

King Hezekiah - II Chronicle 32:26 "Notwithstanding Hezekiah humbled himself for the **pride of his heart**, both he and the inhabitants of Jerusalem, so that the wrath of the LORD came not upon them in the days of Hezekiah."

Moab – Jeremiah 48:29, "We have heard the **pride of Moab**, (he is exceeding proud) his loftiness, and his arrogance, and his pride, and the haughtiness of his heart."

PSYCHOLOGICAL POINT OF VIEW

Psychological point of view is another angle where pride can be explains so we can create a vivid picture of pride and how it affects our spiritual and physical behavior. It is going to be explain in two ways:

Behavioral point of view:

This is a self inflicted behavior that comes as a result of improper learning, arrogant, ignorant and lack of adequate knowledge of a purpose. The behavioral point of view states that pride is wrongly learnt and applied in our everyday life. It is wrongly learned because of people we make our model. The books we read sometime can misinterpret pride as a normal variable of life. Healthy form of pride that acknowledges God in its totality is not dangerous but when the presences of God begin to extinct and fade away gradually. Yes, this is because pride is not a day or week process, it is an unconscious development that seems right in the sight of the individual but overtime deadly.

Psychoanalytical Point of View:

Pride in this context is described as abnormal behavior which is a result of imbalance between the three major components or internal drives namely: (1) the id (2) the ego and (3) super ego. The id which I consider to be the flesh (seeks to gratify its desire at all cost not minding the side effect), a motivating or propelling or instinctual drive that is lustful, desiring personal attributions, self centered, selfish and seek immediate gratification of desire regardless of the consequences. From Freud explanation, it is believed that pride victims have an inflated ego or under developed ego, that is why you see pride victim personifying themselves. Freud concluded that some of the powerful influences such as pride, pomposity..... on human personality are things we are not conscious of, hence, it is possible to say that pride victims may not be aware that they are suffering from pride.

Psychoanalytical explanation of pride in this context may not be too Christian-like as some theorists will put it, but it has strong correlation with spiritual explanation. The bible explains that human being is a combination of flesh (id – the selfish drive), soul (ego) and spirit (super ego) which live by societal and spiritual rules. A clear characteristic of these component can further be explain as follow- the man who is spiritually-led go after spiritual things or walk in the spirit, that is the function of the super ego (Morality) **Galatians 5:22-23, 25**. The man who lust after the things of the flesh, usually operates in the flesh, a clear description of the id (lustful) **Galatians 5:18-19**. The ego is our mind; it judges us of our actions. Our minds decides who occupies it, it is either occupy by the spirit of God or the devil. Our mind plays a vital role in harmonizing our body, soul and spirit to unity. Have you ever been judged by what you do. Do you still feel guilty even without the presence of others in such a manner that you cannot sleep? That is the function of the middle man (Ego). You must develop it to tell you the truth in all circumstances, and at all time. This positive development can be done through development of positive attitude of persistence prayer (II Thess. 5:17), renewing your mindset with good virtues, Philippians 4:8, learn to be of good comfort, be of one mind, live in peace, James 1:8, Draw nigh to God, and he will draw nigh to you. Cleanse your hands, and purify your hearts, avoid double minded syndrome.

> ## ➢ HOW DO WE IDENTIFY PRIDE?

Before I go further I wish to say that *self esteem*, and *pride*, should not be misunderstood and see one as the other. In self concept according to Benjamin B. Lahey (2002), it is a subjective of who we are and what we are like, it is an inner directed believe which all people possess that lead them to grow and improve. It does not puff, boast and manifest self centeredness. The self here thought emphasize on the first person pronoun "I" but does not get to his head such that he neglects the presence of a supreme being. They usually make comment like, I know that I can make it because my God liveth, I refuse to give up and fail for God has not given me the spirit of fear, failure and death. You see whatever they say; they acknowledge the presence of God, who is the secrets to their success. The fact that you believe in yourself does not make it a pride but when it become excessively abnormal and self centered.

But in the case of pride, the individual attribute all success to himself and refused to acknowledge the source. He becomes self center and selfish. Pride goeth before destruction (Proverbs 16:18) meaning it is usually ahead of us and blinds us not to see the pit and danger ahead of us.

Let's see how pride manifests itself:
1. **Self Justification**: They rationalized their own attitude and behaviors. Everything they do seem to be right. They

hardly accept mistakes. They easily resort to defense mechanism, unrealistic effort to discharge tension or reality such as reaction formation, denial, anger, bitterness and many more. They are easily frustrated and react negatively and uncontrollably as soon as they are faced with real life situation.

2. They manifest **narcissistic personality disorder** - an unrealistic sense of self important preoccupied fantasies of future success; requiring constant attention and praise, lack genuine concern for others, emphasis is usually on the self. They will always want to be notice in any situation.

3. Pride has another form, look around you, there are some who hardly talk or associate with others, not that they do not want to talk or associate with others. They feel, think and see others as inferior to them. Something I called **pride like humility.** It is just the sense of pride that makes them see others as inferiors.

Hence, they develop lack of clear conscience for them. I do not like associating myself with these set of people. The reason is that they are not their class. A haughty look, a proud look and the plowing of the wicked are sin (Proverb 21:4).

CONQUERING PRIDE:
The number one step is to identify it is the spiritual approach prayer, thanksgiving and meditation are not only recommended but declares a moment specifically dedicated to fasting and prayer against the spirit of pride.

The second approach is the **psychological therapy: two things are involve in the life of every individual (1) his perception (2) his behavior (emotions and physical actions).** Psychological therapy is an approach that creates awareness and understanding of abnormal behaviors. Awareness is the number one instrument of healing; otherwise any other form of miracle will be in vain. Psychotherapy is all about creating awareness about the unknown and that is why **every man of God is a psychotherapist and every psychotherapist is a man of God**. They are there to help people change for good. After all, what is repentance if it is not all about positive change of behavior? I mean migrating from maladaptive to adaptive behavior, doing what the public, society and heaven consider being good and acceptable. The survival and wellbeing of the society is what we are preaching. We tend to see more of criminal behaviors and neglecting personality disorders as a societal problem.

I once told a friend of mine, instead of organizing revivals in the name financial, healing and miracle for sale display, why not see it as a medium for behavioral changes and he look at me with a smile. Many seek miracle at all cost, instead of changing the individual mindset for good, restructure his mentality for positive thinking, we are so concern about healing, money, blessings. Mean while sin is in the increase, with many false men of god enriching their pockets through technical and structural extortion from blessing and miracle seekers.

Most victims of pride are not even aware of the fact that pride is in them. One may ask, what is psychology got to do with spiritual matters? The answer is simply "Yes." Psychology is designed to help create awareness about the reality of life, replace maladaptive behaviors with adaptable or acceptable form of behaviors, the one we all call "**sin**". What is the difference between repentance and behavioral modification if I may ask? Is it not changing from evil to good, rejecting what is bad and accepting what is right and doing what is right? Psychology is concern with the mindset, creating awareness about your limitations, gifts, talents, what you can and what you cannot do, management of resources, understanding of the self toward spiritual and physical growth.

Introspection; According to Coleman (2003) defines it as a method of data collection in which observers record and describe their own internal mental and physical experiences. In other words, introspection has to do with examination of the self. It requires a self evaluation. Questions like I am doing the right thing? is my life in line with God's standard and humanity. These questions have personal explanations rather than external answers. Introspection has to do with your personal evaluation and assessment as well as personal reward which include success and/or failure, blames and praises. Whichever way, the individual will know the truth and stands the chance to either correct mistakes, adjust some abnormalities, remove or unlearn some abnormal facts, learn new behaviors and/or reinforce successful ones.

The relevance of introspection therefore, helps us to look backward to see where we are coming, where we are and where we are going to. In other words, you can see the past obstacles, acknowledge the present and have an insight of the future. I think it should be a mistake to deny the past. You can learn from other people's mistake but most importantly is the mistake of the person himself. The reason is this, you only know that the other person made mistake but you may not know what he did that prompted his mistakes or failure, but you will learn very well from your mistake because you will know what you did or what you did not do that resulted to your mistakes or success. Introspection therefore is a process of having proper reflection of the past.

CHAPTER 10
HEALING THE MIND

"Our minds is the womb for great ideal of success or failure, the wall within which this success or failure is nurtured"

A writer once said Those who exert the first influence upon the mind, have the greatest power. The psychology of the human mind try to pin point ways by which we can manage and direct the thoughts produced by our minds. Our minds is such an important aspect of our existence as well as well being where great ideas are manufacture, achievement, dreams, sense of optimism, aspiration, and visions for spiritual and physical transformation are built upon. It is only those who understand this hiding concept and apply same to the demand of life that truly enjoys life to its fullest. One thing you must understand about your mind is that it could either be occupied by the spirit of God or Satan.

SRI AUROBINDO once said there is nothing the mind can do that cannot be better done in the mind's immobility and thought-free stillness. It functions are directed by who reside in it. That is the reason the Bible described the human behavior (overt or covert) through the structure of his mind. The spirit of God in one's mind radiates the following fruits: joy, love, hopefulness, positive focus, Godly wisdom, peace and stability of the mind and soul, gentility, full of mercy and Meekness, temperance, without partiality, and without hypocrisy.

Evil thoughts on the other hand, are the products of satanic control. These People see nothing about themselves and the future. These set of human being are characterized by internal sickness of the mind. Something psychoanalyst called intra psyches conflict. These people are characterized by lack of connection or balance between their real self and the reality of life. They are riddles with very poor sense of judgment about themselves and life generally. They are filled with negative ideations, pessimism, discouragement, hopelessness, self unbelief, doubt, self limitation, self denial, paralyzed mental state, confusion about the beauty and reality of life, rejection, depressed to the point of death and in most cases followed by sense of suicide. The most dangerous aspect of these negative characteristics of unhealthy mind is that it is unconsciously transmittable and infectious. Sick minded people are barrier to societal growth and development. They affect others by discouraging and paralyzing those healthy minds.

WHAT TO DO

Since our minds are such an important aspect of our existence. We must therefore be guided by certain principles of doing the right thing. Our minds speak through our mouths and see more than our eyes can see. Our minds first act before our sense organs respond.

Proverbs 12: 20-23 "Deceit is in the heart(mind) of them that imagine evil: but to the counsellors of peace is joy. A prudent man concealeth knowledge: but the heart(mind) of fools proclaimeth foolishness."

My mind changes often ... People who have no mind can easily be steadfast and firm, but when a man is loaded down to the guards with it, as I am, every heavy sea of foreboding or inclination, maybe of indolence, shifts the cargo. **MARK TWAIN, letter to James Redpath, Aug. 8, 1871**

Cognitive psychologists believe most people are psychologically sick and behave abnormally because of negative thoughts, reasoning that are incorporate into their minds. According to Psychoanalysts, any individual with intra psyches conflict is a sick individual who lack confidence in himself. Humanistic psychologists believe such an individual has a severe disintegrated self concept and will continue to experience an imbalance state of mind until he comes to himself in one piece.

SELF DISCOVERY: Self discovery is coming to term with your real self and the reality of God's purpose. God created you. He endowed you with talents and potentials. You make yourself who you are. You maximize your talents and potentials. Who you are is the product of what you make yourself. The process of making yourself who you are is the fulfillment of what God created you to be. This can best be fulfilled by self discovery. Self discovery is the first tool you need to start the journey of success, greatness and spiritual wellness and growth. Without proper discovery of the self, any struggle of life simply means that you are operating in the shadow of another man's destiny. In self discovery, you must bring into reality your strength and weakness. You must as well find out your core potentials that truly define your real self. Many are alive yet operating in another's man destiny. This is the worst error of life- living the dream of another person.

SELF EVALUATION: When John the beloved was talking in III John 1:2, that he wishes above all things that you may prosper and be in health, even as thy soul prospers". He was given his readers a powerful means of self evaluation that has to do with more than just physical prosperity but spiritual wellness based on God's way of life. John the beloved was trying to give us a picture of spiritual wellness through a methodical introspection which is much more than the physical prosperity or worldly acquisition of materialism.

SELF ACCEPTANCE: There is huge different from **breaking from your pseudo personality** and **accepting your true self**. When you break from pseudo personality, you break from limitations that prevents you from been your real self but when you accept your real self, it gives you the boldness to be the very person that you are and potentially moving toward your destiny. Very many people want to be like the other person. The fact that Bishop T.D. Jakes is your mentor or hero does not make you Bishop T.D. Jakes. I have heard a lot of people saying "I wish I had your brain (wisdom). I wish I was like the other person. You are unique and peculiar from any human being on earth. I Peter 2:9 say "But ye are a **chosen generation**, a **royal priesthood**, a holy nation, a **peculiar** people; that ye should shew forth the praises of him who hath called you out of darkness into his marvelous light". This is the secret behind the above verse:

A Chosen Generation: It reminds us that we are a special linage of God's representatives on earth. We carried the genetic blue-print of God's attributes. We are specially figured out among the crowed to bear the characteristic of Christ Jesus. When God said let us make man in our own image and likeness in Genesis 1:26 he created us to function like him, we should be able to say, let there be and it will come to pass. Jesus Christ did not come to give us a new creation, God has already created us, he only come to redeem and restore us back to the father's original purpose of creation.

A Royal Priesthood: This signifies God's magnificent leadership. It denotes that you are a God's head. Nobody on earth will ever function and reason likes you. That is why when you are not there things will either slow down or cease to function. A priest is an intercessor. If you are a priest then you are that person who will always plead for the cause of others. You must see less of yourself and focus much on the welfare and goodness of others. You must pray for the spiritual welfare of others much more than your physical and spiritual welfare. Exodus 19:6 says "And ye shall be unto me a kingdom of priests, and a holy nation. These are the words which thou shalt speak unto the children of Israel". You do not curse people but bless them with a holy prayer to God. Until you discover yourself as a priest, you will continue to live in the shadow of emptiness.

A Holy Nation: It signifies that you are among the Godly elected or representatives that are consecrated for his majestic purpose. You are not just a nation but a Holy

Nation. You are just like one among the twenty four elders in Heaven singing saying "Holy, Holy, Holy, is the LORD of hosts: the whole earth is full of his glory" Isaiah 6:3. While the twenty four elders are in heaven glorifying God, you are on earth magnifying and giving him praises.

A Peculiar Person: Peculiarity is the only attribute that makes you matchless in this world. You are so unique, matchless, exclusive, gloriously designed, outstanding and exceptional in all things. Have you ever asked yourself, why do people envy me? The answer is simple; they see something inside you that you do not even see. When the Psalmist discovered this amazing grace, he said "**What is man (who is me)**, that thou art mindful of him? and the son of man, that thou visitest him?" A peculiar person means you more than just an ordinary being. You are perfected or created for a special purpose. There is nobody that can function like you and there will be no other person on earth that will function and fit into your peculiarity even ten thousand years after you are gone from this planet earth.

Show Forth the Praises (Fruitfulness): There is one thing very many persons are yet to discover about themselves. You may be greenish (beautiful or handsome), you will only look like a beautiful tree without fruits to show. Fruitfulness is not just physical attainments of worldly materialism but that attainment level of spiritual growth, development and fruitfulness that glorifies God. In Isaiah 43:7, He said "**I created you for my glory**..." Matthew 7:20 concluded by saying "wherefore by their fruits ye shall know them".

SELF EMPOWERMENT: Your ability to develop the "I can do it mentality" is something many are yet to discovered. The very best gift you can give yourself is to empower your life never to call it a quit no matter what happens in life. Philippians 4:18 says but **I have all**, and **abound**: **I am full**, ... to God. Can you see the three key words here; "**I HAVE**", "**ABOUND**" and "I **AM**

FULL". Until you learn how to motivate yourself, encourage your inner man to go further, and the ability to never call it a quit, things will never change. My father died when I was eleven, just a week to my twelfth birthday. My mother had nothing to offer other than moral advise and encouragement, but today, I have written books that many have discovered their places in life and many others writings coming up.

SELF REPOSITIONING: Every radio or television station has frequency upon which it operates. There will be scrabbling until the proper frequency is met. This is applicable to man. Until your mind and mentality is reposition to see connect to term with life's reality, you will remain where you are and will amount to nothing in life. **You were not created for nothing but something**. You were created for a purpose and for the glory of God. Even every one that is called by my name: for I have created him for my glory, I have formed him; yea, I have made him, (Isaiah 43:7).

Put your trust in Him (God through Jesus Christ) John 14:6 "I am the way, the truth and the way, no one come to the father except by me". John 1:12 says "But as **many as received him**, to them **gave HE power** to **become the sons of God**, even to them that **believe on his name". This is an absolute act of Divine transformation.** According as his divine power hath given unto us all things that pertain unto life and godliness, through the knowledge of him that hath called us to glory and virtue: Whereby are given unto us **exceeding great** and **precious promises**: that by these ye might be **partakers of the divine nature**, having escaped the corruption that is in the world through lust.

The Connection: Our behaviors are majorly affected and influenced by incoming sensory variables. The people around you influence you, your learning processes influence you, the books read influence you, and the people you associate with also play such a vital role in what you become. At this point you should ask yourself questions like

- ✓ Who are these people around me?
- ✓ How are they influencing my life?
- ✓ Where are I am going?
- ✓ What will I be twenty years to come?
- ✓ What can I do to design the future to my favor?

Philippians 4:8 then summarized it all by saying "Finally, brethren, whatsoever things are true, whatsoever things are honest, whatsoever things are just, whatsoever things are pure, whatsoever things are lovely, whatsoever things are of good report; if there be any virtue, and if there be any praise, think on these things".

The world is place of connected gifts. Every gifted person has his/her gift connected to others. We play vital roles in the fulfillment of other people's destiny. If you cripple yourself, you will paralyze more than thousands gifts out there. It is what you do that makes the different. First thing to note is by breaking out of your limitation and comfort zone. There are amazing and beautiful things of life that you have not seen. They are all yours if you step out of faith. The best way to prove your mind is by programming your mind to see thing clearly in the mind. You also have to transform those things you see in your mind and begin to make them take the form of reality.

You must train your mind to hold on to integrity, honesty and self discipline. Until you begin to convert the things your mind see to reality, you will forever remain a dreamer. It is good to dream but it is abnormal to remain a dreamer. Dreamers are always in a world of delusional fantasies of greatness. Genesis 13:3 says "thou shall not hearken unto the words of that prophet, or that **dreamer of dreams**: for the LORD your God prove you, to know whether ye love the LORD your God with all your heart and with all your soul". These possibilities start from the mind. Our minds are the starting point toward our success or failures.

ENVISION GREATNESS: The entire world is divided into two groups of persons. This includes those who see with their eyes and those who see minds. Those who see with eyes, see today. Those who see with minds, see the future. The future is like the depth of the ocean. It takes diverse to go beyond the ordinary. There are things beyond what we see that can best be seen with our minds. Deuteronomy 29:29 says "The **secret things** of nature (80%) belong unto the LORD our God: but those things which are revealed (20%) belong unto us and to our children for ever, that we may do all the words of this law". Daniel 2:19 and 22, put it this way, "Then was the secret revealed unto Daniel in a night vision." Then Daniel blessed the God of heaven. "He (God) reveals the deep and secret things: he knows what is in the darkness, and the light dwell with him." When the Psalmist discovered this secret, he said blessed is he that delight in the law of the Lord and meditate (Putting your whole mind) in the things of God. I earlier told you that the mind is cosmic and transcend to the unseen heavenly place. You must therefore program your mind to operate at that level of life. Proverb 1:5 says "A wise man will hear, and will increase in learning; and a man of understanding shall attain unto wise counsels". Isaiah said, **learn to do good**. Isaiah went further to say in 29:11, and the vision of all is become unto you as the words of a book that is sealed, **which men deliver to one that is learned**, saying, read this, I pray thee: and he said, I cannot; for it is sealed.

You must train and position your mind to see good things in the future. Even in the midst of hopeless and critical situation, Brother Job still declared "I know my redeemer liveth". Isaiah said let your soul and mind delight in fatness of life. A healthy man is the product of a healthy mind that sees a beautiful feature.

CHAPTER 11
A MOMENT OF SOBER REFLECTION

Man will have to acknowledge one basic fact that he is a product of a hand work, Genesis 1; 26- "man made in his image," Isaiah 43:7- "man was created for God's glory." Jeremiah 18:4-6 ssaid "God designed man to suit his purpose." More so, man is a finite being while God is an infinite being. Man needs the presence of God to gain true joy and lasting peace. Until this is realized, the gap between him and his creator will continue to erode. Man will continue to languish in pain and regrets. Like I earlier said, we needs to realize that we are creations and that there is a creator (God) who owns everything about us. Man's **spiritual growth and success** depends largely on the extents of his relationship with his creator. As Christians, we need to realize the very purpose for our creation and not on the basis of experiment, evolution or chances as some theorists put it.

In Isaiah 43:7 "every one that is **called by my name**; for I have created Him for my Glory, I have formed him; yea I have made Him." In Deuteronomy 8:18- "But thou shall remember the lord your God, for it is **HE** that giveth thee **power to acquire wealth**. So the possibility to succeed lies largely on the extent of the relationship between you and your creator. The above passages simply remind us of a **higher authority**. There is no way in which you can successfully boast of making it in life without the presence of God. The truth is real Christians do not struggle for food, happiness and lasting peace because all these belong to their father.

We are made in **God likeness** and his image and that God having the will-power also deposited this **will-power** in us to make decisions, Deuteronomy 30:15 see, **I have set before thee this day life and good, and death and evil**. The will-power empowers us to make and enforce decisions. It is therefore, imperative to say that the decision to either fail or success depend entirely on how we manifest this will-power. The **presence of God** will continue to remind us of who we are, that is why we need Him. The basic question in life is who am I, what can I do, what are my capabilities and talents in life, what are my limitations? Of course we have **limitations in life**; where am I coming from and where am I going to, am I a product of evolution, chance or probability, or some kind of **experimental exercises** or what else, if I am not a product of evolution or experiment, then why was I created in the first instance? Why was I not born two hundred years ago or may be a thousand years ago, why now, why this very moment? May be there is a purpose for this.

I think this call for a moment of sober reflection, a food for thought and demonstration of the true nature of which we are, and the very reason for our creation. This reminds me of the preacher in **Ecclesiastes 6:3**- "if a man lives a hundred years, and live many years, so that the days of his years are many, but he does not **enjoy** life's good things and also has no burial, I say that untimely birth is better off than he." This portion of the Bible just gave me a message about the early life and death of **Jesus Christ** who lived only thirty three years on earth yet fulfilled his Divine mission. I think the basic question we should ask ourselves is this, what will people say of me when I am long gone? Will I be remembered for **evil or good**, will they remember my name at all, will my name continue to make an impact or will my name die with me?

This question can only be answered when the individual discover who he is, that he begin to discover himself, where is coming from and where he is going to, exploits the potentials around him. When the Angel asked Jacob what is your name, he replied Jacob, the Angel said no wonder. Jacob never knew who he was until his confrontation with angel of God. And I believed by God's supernatural power any one reading this message will discover the true purpose for his life in the name of Jesus Christ, amen.

The truth is this; many have not discovered who they are, their potentials and what they can do. Those who have discovered themselves are bound in ignorance and are in the wrong path of life so they fight for a wrong cause. They wrestle in darkness, pains, futility, and failure, simply because they have not found themselves on the right path which is Jesus Christ- the way, the truth and light to success(John 14:6) .

I think it is time we ask and answer these questions ourselves.

1) Who are my?
2) Am I a product of chance, evolution or creation?
3) Is my life subject to a living God or something else or nothing at all?
4) If with God, then is my relationship with God cordial, loose or not at all?
5) Is the bible true word of God or just a write up?
6) What of all the promises contained in it?

7) Is my life on the right path and purpose of my creation?

8) Can I do it alone or do I need the help of God or god?

9) What will happen after I am long gone?

10) Is there life after death or everything ends here?

11) Is there any name like Jesus or is it a name like any other great men mentioned in books and other historical records?

12) What is the true meaning of the name-Jesus?

13) How powerful is that name- Jesus, or is it the preconceived notions of our minds that the name Jesus seem so powerful?

14) Why will I be so conscious of a name that I have never seen?

15) Am I truly in lines with God commandments mentioned in the bible?

THINGS YOU MUST UNDERSTAND ABOUT PRAYER

(a) Prayer must be consistence, see II Thessalonians 5:16-17; pray without ceasing......... do not quench the spirit. It means that when you stop praying, you starve you spiritual being.

(b) Prayer must be seen as part of the individual's life. It must not been seen as a timely practice.

(c) Prayer must be made holy and sanctified.

(d) Prayer must not be insincere and deceitful. Anyway, no man can deceive, God (Gal 6:7).

(e) Prayer is by no mean the most powerful instrument of healing, and sound health. Prayer connects with you with God, so you can make your personal need. Prayer connects you to the source of your success. It is the only medium through which you can connect the owner of success, the provider of wealth and health. Prayer helps you activates what seems like dream to reality. Your ability and commitment to prayer is the only spiritual root to prosperity and good health.

(f) Prayer must not be said on selfish bases. God gives generously to them that ask in sincerity James 1:5, but to those with selfish desire he will not answer- James 4:1-4.

(g) Avoid the use of die, die philosophy or excessive repetitions in your prayer. Jesus Christ never though us that pattern of prayer. God is not deaf. He hears us perfectly well. If at all, you want to use it which of course may not be wrong, should be used on demonic agents who are mortal beings witches and wizards. For the devil himself and his angel cannot die now. There is an appointed time for the devil and his angel of darkness. The bible only said suffers not a witch to live and not the devil to live.

(h) Prayer must be made with humility, sanctity and reverend. For God is pure and Holy, therefore, those coming in his presence must come Holy, in spirit and truth (John 4:24).

THE WAY OUT

The first thing is to totally acknowledge him in all we do. A man cannot say God is God when he lacks the true conviction that Jesus Christ is the true son of God and God all the treasures of life belong to him. That is the reason those without this true conviction run to place without guarantee of lasting blessing of riches and treasure. A place where after a short while you will be asked to forfeit all that you enjoyed with your life and even that of others.

Abiding in the presence of God for just an hour brings an **unending joy** and consecrates our lives to him. Mind you, it is he who gives you the power to acquire wealth and power.

Make God your prime focus in all you do. Until we learn how to fully put our commitments and make Him first in everything we do, we will continue to experience pain, run in futile and regrets. We must therefore be ready to apply the abiding principle, making God our foundation and pillar of success. We can only do this when we have the accurate knowledge of him through fervent studying and meditation of the bible on daily bases. If we are not ready to apply the abiding principle, then true success should not be our focus. Just as Christ rightly said it, if you abide in me and my words in you, you will ask anything in my father's name and it shall granted unto you-John 15:5-7.

Your mind is your airport to the anywhere in the universe. According to HERMANN HESSE "the mind is international and supra-national ... it ought to serve not war and annihilation, but peace and reconciliation." With your mind, you can see the entire world in just one place called the mind. But you must first train, reposition and feed it with the require ingredients of life.

Life is a variety. What you dislike, another person appreciates. What you ignore is treasured by another person. Everything about life is beautiful, adorable and well designed for a purpose. God so designed the things of life base on its season and reasons. That is the reason everything happens at a specified time. The problem is that we only designed or program our mind to hate some, dislike and/or like others. The food you hate is cherished by somebody. Life is like a pie chart. You cannot be found in all the sectors of life at a time. Our inabilities to meet with the challenges of life then subject our mind toward many directions and as a result confused our mind on which way to go. We often talked about the wandering mind but we never ask why the wandering mind. The wondering mind is first of all a confused mind. A confused mind on the other hand is a burden mind of restlessness, lost direction and a wrong purpose for life. Until this very purpose and direction is rediscovery it will be a hard way drive to a healthy and successful mind.

Karl Marx once said "the true power of the mind, its impact on our health, future, outlook, and self-concept, is a mystery, sparking much discussion and debate for centuries. As food for thought, here's what some of the world's most respected figures of the past along with some of today's most recognized inspirational speakers and writers, have to offer on this intriguing subject. " This is one of my favorite quotes because it gives me the power to annex the power of mind mostly when I am getting depress and spiritually weak. It reawakens my mind to boldness.

Jim Rohn reminds me that each time I start thinking and saying what I really want my mind automatically shifts and pulls push me in that direction. Martin Luther King has this to say as long as the mind is enslaved; the body can never be free. Psychological freedom is a firm sense of self-esteem, is the most powerful weapon against the long night of physical slavery.

Every human being is born original, unique and peculiar yet many die photocopy. Don't live the life of another man.

You are what you are by becoming what you want to become. Nobody can stop you becoming who you are until you stop yourself from being what you are.

Your mind controls your body; never allow your body controls your mind. Your mind is your life; your life is controlled by what your mind dictates.

www.ingramcontent.com/pod-product-compliance
Lightning Source LLC
Chambersburg PA
CBHW072122280526
45788CB00002B/513